THE CHILD'S DISCOVERY OF DEATH

Founded by C. K. Ogden

The International Library of Psychology

DEVELOPMENTAL PSYCHOLOGY
In 32 Volumes

THE CHILD'S DISCOVERY OF DEATH

A Study in Child Psychology

SYLVIA ANTHONY

Introduction by J C Flugel

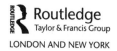

Routledge
Taylor & Francis Group
LONDON AND NEW YORK

First published in 1940 by
Routledge

Reprinted in 1999 by
Routledge
2 Park Square, Milton Park, Abingdon, Oxon, OX14 4RN

Simultaneously published in the USA and Canada by Routledge

711 Third Avenue, New York, NY 10017

Transferred to Digital Printing 2007

Routledge is an imprint of the Taylor & Francis Group, an informa business

First issued in paperback 2013

© 1940 Sylvia Anthony

The publishers have made every effort to contact authors/copyright holders
of the works reprinted in the *International Library of Psychology*.
This has not been possible in every case, however, and we would
welcome correspondence from those individuals/companies
we have been unable to trace.

These reprints are taken from original copies of each book. In many cases
the condition of these originals is not perfect. The publisher has gone to
great lengths to ensure the quality of these reprints, but wishes to point
out that certain characteristics of the original copies will, of necessity, be
apparent in reprints thereof.

British Library Cataloguing in Publication Data
A CIP catalogue record for this book
is available from the British Library

The Child's Discovery of Death
ISBN 978-0-415-20981-6 (hbk)
ISBN 978-0-415-86438-1 (pbk)

Dedicated
with love, faith and hope
to
Charles
Daniel
David
Elizabeth
Jenneth
Joanna
Paul and
William

June, 1940

CONTENTS

INTRODUCTION

By Professor J. C. Flugel

Most of us appear willing to accept with complacency the general characteristics of living matter—the spontaneity and relative unpredictability of its movement and the complex metabolic processes that underlie this movement. Being made of living matter ourselves, our prime business is to live, and it requires a fairly high degree of sophistication before our curiosity is aroused as to just what is involved in living, as to what is the essential difference between living and non-living things. To this general tendency to take the processes and peculiarities of living for granted there are two striking exceptions. Living organisms die and they reproduce, and these two aspects of life exercise upon us an uncanny fascination. The fact that, after a certain time or in consequence of certain misadventures, the individual organism ceases to display the characteristics of living and tends to disintegrate ; the other fact that, following on certain actions on the part of living organisms, new living beings come into existence—these facts have for us a disturbing, indeed often an overwhelming, significance, whether we contemplate them as mere occurrences in the outer world or experience them as having, actually or potentially, an intimate relation to ourselves. The existence even of large and highly complex living creatures we are prepared to accept without astonishment, our curiosity being aroused only by some (to us) unusual feature of size, structure or behaviour. But that these large and complex beings should have a beginning and an end : these are facts to which our interest and attention seem to be naturally attuned, and which tend to arouse both intellectual activity and emotional upheaval—more particularly when the beings concerned belong to our own species, and most of all when they form part of our own close and intimate environment.

In human societies these interests and emotions are often, perhaps always, institutionalized. Anthropology has shown that, among primitive peoples all over the earth, birth and death and all that appertains to them are the occasions of innumerable ritual observances and the subjects of vast systems of superstitious belief. On the one hand, we have the widespread and varied puberty rites and initiation ceremonies, marriage ceremonies, taboos and rituals with regard to copulation, still others affecting menstruation, the practices connected with birth itself, and finally the weird but again widespread natal and post-natal procedures involved in the Couvade. On the other hand, we find an obstinate refusal to accept the fact of natural death and an elaborate structure of magical belief and practice designed to bolster up this refusal—a magic which itself contains the beginnings of the healing art and of the science of medicine ; we find, too, the complicated development of funerary rites and sacrifices, and an even greater elaboration of theories concerning the existence of a life after death and what happens in that life. Furthermore, through the belief in reincarnation and rebirth, a bridge is formed between the two sets of phenomena, which thus become interrelated and perhaps eventually incorporated in a single metaphysical system.

Modern psychology (especially that of the psycho-analytic school) has in its turn shown that birth and death are no less significant to our own society and to the individuals that compose it. No matter how much or how little we accept the particular theories of psycho-analysts or of the other psychologists who have concerned themselves with sex, we all of us believe to-day that sexual problems and the way in which they are solved have some very real importance for the development and mental health of the individual. Hence the great number of books on the psychology of sex that have appeared in recent years, including many that deal with the impact of sexual ideas and experiences on the mind of the child and the practical problems to which this impact may give rise.

There is no corresponding literature on the psychology of death—and this in spite of the fact that psycho-analysis has shown that in many important respects our attitude towards death is similar to that towards sex. Both subjects are often unpleasant, inasmuch as they tend to arouse anxiety (though at bottom the anxiety may be differently motivated) ; we often react to both forms of unpleasure and anxiety by the same devices of flight, repression, taboo and symbolism (we talk of a " departed " friend as we talk of a " fallen " woman, shunning in both cases the greater affect that a more direct expression might involve) ; both subjects may be intimately bound together in ideas of widespread or indeed of universal significance, as in the Œdipus complex ; and there has been found in the individual mind the same curious and somewhat mystic relationship between the ideas of birth and death that is revealed in so many of the social beliefs brought to light by the anthropologist or the student of comparative religion. It is clear that the subject of death has not merited this relative neglect, and that the impact on the individual mind, especially the immature mind, of the idea of death, the ways in which the mind attempts to deal with this disturbing subject, and the theories which are formed in the course of this attempt, are quite as worthy of study as are the corresponding processes in the field of sex and reproduction. It is to just such a study that the present book is devoted. Now that it lies before us, it seems evident that such a book is considerably overdue. Sylvia Anthony is to be congratulated on having had the courage to overcome the resistances and taboos which have hitherto surrounded this difficult and delicate subject—a courage comparable to that of the writers who braved the corresponding sexual taboos a decade or two ago.

But the book is not merely overdue ; it has a certain grim appropriateness to the present time, when we have perforce to familiarize ourselves with the idea of death, imminent for us, for those about us, or those dear to us. Writing twenty-five years ago, during the last great war, Freud in his memorable essay, *Thoughts for the Times on War and Death,* warned us with characteristic realism that in this matter, as in others with which he had previously dealt, we were tending to live psychologically beyond our means, and that it might be well for us to realize more fully the true nature of our attitude towards death—an attitude that we are only too willing to distort or suppress to save our own or others' feelings. Now that we are in the throes of another mighty conflict, it is more than ever incumbent upon us to take this warning to heart. To deal frankly with the psychology of death, he said (as he had already told us in the case of sex), " has the merit of taking somewhat more into account the true state of affairs, and of making life again more endurable for us." With this courageous and deeply realistic aim of making life more endurable, let us turn with all due gratitude to the illuminating study that Sylvia Anthony has here provided.

PREFACE

THE study on which this book is based was planned in 1937 and completed early in 1939. It is a psychological study. It aims at contributing to the establishment of general laws of human development.

All the subjects of the study are English children, contemporaries of one another. Their thoughts and emotions and forms of expression have been moulded by the culture and the age in which they live. The material is therefore sociologically limited. Can general psychological conclusions validly be drawn from it?

I am far from thinking that Death is a manifestation of " external reality " which presents itself similarly to every " normal " child in the course of his development. I believe that many aspects of the culture that surrounded these children influenced their ideas of death and the way they came to discover the fact of it.

All psychological law of general significance requires what may be briefly called *correction for relevant context* before it can be applied in any individual case. To determine what is relevant context is a main part of the search for psychological law.

As this study progressed it appeared that the aspects of culture (the sociological context) relevant to laws of the development of the idea of death in children were certain fundamental attitudes held, in the main, in common all over the civilized world. But the term " civilized " is of disputable application. I mean that part of human society in which the heritage of Palestine and Hellas is cherished and fruitful.

From this it would follow that although the conclusions drawn from this material are not necessarily applicable as they stand to the mental development of every human child, they should, if they are sound, prove valid for the great majority of children reared in the same culture, when the word is used in this wide sense. Since the present material is so homogeneous, this claim can easily be tested, and I hope it will be.

Even within this comparatively homogeneous English scene, sociological distinctions existed, of social class, urban and rural life, forms of religion, and so on. Contrary to expectation, no perceptible differences were found to result from these, in the children's reactions. That is not to say that a study specially designed to discover such differences in children's ideas of death would fail to discover any ; only, that in a study not planned for this particular purpose, such differences form a comparatively insignificant part of the general pattern of mental development.

Although, looking back, men may see this period as part of an interval between two great wars, the lives and thoughts of English children were not, I believe, affected by war, during the months when this study was made, any more than is normal for children in democratic countries during the intervals of peace. Their behaviour, indeed, may in respect of the idea of death provide a standard against which those caring for children in war-time may roughly measure their reactions under unaccustomed stresses.

I believe they will find that in war-time it is not so much aspects of death previously unrealized which distress the child, as the changing of life-patterns in which his emotions have been anchored. Thus a little girl accused of stealing from her billet-mother told me, " When my father told our John he was going in the army, he (John) started to cry." " Why ? " " 'Cos he wanted him to stop with my mother." It is from complex miseries such as this that most childish neuroses in war-time arise.

War and its demands fill our minds to-day. But experiences of alarm, danger and utmost horror or grief appear to precipitate rather than initiate mental instability or disorder. Reactions in childhood to the idea of death, on the other hand, may lie at the very root of such morbid development. In the connections between the two, an immense field lies open for exploration, almost untrodden. This study lies only at the gateway ; yet it seemed to me that from this position one had a view of new scientific riches and new hopes for human happiness that lay beyond.

I could not have undertaken this work without the help of many friends and members of my family. First of all, I must thank those parents who have, over a considerable period of time, kept special records for me of their children's sayings and behaviour, many of which are transcribed in the text. I wish I could thank them by name, but that cannot be. Mrs. Norman, until the outbreak of war Senior Psychologist at Guy's Hospital, first drew my attention to the Geneva Story-Completion Test, and in many other ways gave me assistance for which no mere acknowledgment is adequate recognition. Through her application permission was granted to me, as a student at Guy's (in the Department of Psychological Medicine), to work in schools under the London County Council where the head teacher was also willing to give permission ; to these head teachers I would also express my gratitude. The country children I was able to study through the kindness of my husband's cousin, the Revd. Cuthbert Holden. Although the material has been treated statistically only at one point, some problems arose in that connection which I could scarcely have solved without the help of Mr. A. T. Marshall and Mr. Babington-Smith. Professor J. C. Flugel supervised the original study from beginning to end. His supervision not only prevented innumerable faults and omissions from appearing in the text, but meant much more than that : suggestions of unnoted aspects of the subject, and unwearied encouragement. Indeed, I once went to him with the proposal that the whole study should be abandoned because nothing of any value could come of it, and it was only his dissuasion, his tentative hopefulness that some result might be achieved, which impelled me to continue. I should add that I alone must be held responsible for omissions and faults in the text, and also, that the beginning and end of the present work were written after the original study, and so have not received the same helpful criticism as the rest. Finally, I have to thank my father, who has given me £50 for three years so that I could undertake psychological research. Obviously the final outcome must owe much more to him than that, but the other things cannot be so easily measured. He has not read a word of the text, nor have we met since long before the work was planned, but I should find it hard to say for what he is *not* responsible.

CHAPTER I

THIS study, first undertaken as a piece of research into the mental development of children, has gained deeper topical significance from events occurring as its last words are written. In this and other countries millions of young children have been separated from their parents and taken away to other billets. As the imminence of danger fluctuates, families in each country are separated or re-united. In many countries of Europe now, young children's fathers are under arms, and the shadow of death hangs over the families they come from. The problem of allaying or not arousing childish anxiety used to be mainly the mother's, but now it is shared by many teachers, who are placed more fully in charge of children than they have formerly been. They will have the task of handling psychological situations which cannot but be new to them. For some of the children there will inevitably be grief that has objective cause. There will be individual anxieties, and also those permeations of individual reactions among a group that may issue in panic, or (as sometimes among the Basque refugees) in wild aggressions. There will also be (more subtle to understand, and far more difficult to handle) those griefs, anxieties and irrational aggressions which have no apparent objective cause, but may be signs or precursors of psychoneurotic trouble, hysterical illness, or of anti-social behaviour such as leads to the criminal court.

Such indications of grief and anxiety will occur, and will be recognized by those who have learnt how to recognize

B   1

them. There will also be children who display an apparent lack of "natural" emotional reaction to situations which the adult thinks should normally arouse deep feeling. The child may be considered heartless, or in some other way deficient. In handling such cases, perhaps more than with any others, an understanding of the normal psychological development of children, going somewhat deeper than that usually required of the classroom teacher, is essential. At some stages of child-development, and in some personalities still within the range of the emotionally normal, it is probable that such reactions need not be a source of anxiety to those in charge of the child. At a different stage of development, or in a different personality, they may indicate the beginning of dissociative processes in mental experience—the refusal to accept the bitter thing into the emotional life—which may later culminate in serious disintegration of the mind. Psychiatry is at present almost helpless when certain forms of mental illness have developed so far as to produce typically psychotic behaviour. It may be that schizophrenia, for instance, is preventable or curable, at a stage which is scarcely to be recognized as yet as its incipient form. The present research suggests that closer study of the development of the concept of death in the individual may help to elucidate the origins of certain forms of mental disorder. And, in more immediately practical terms, that if a child with a tendency to react dissociatively (with peculiar lack of "emotional" behaviour) to experiences of death, is handled with psychological insight, or given immediate and suitable psychotherapy when the trouble occurs, a slow process of mental disintegration which might date from that period may be averted.

When psychogenic factors are sought as causes of later mental disorder, stress has mainly been laid on thought-patterns of which sexual impulses are the central activating nucleus (unconscious processes being included in the term *thought*). This view is not necessarily opposed to an interpretation which lays special stress on the reactions to the idea of death, for these reactions have a very close connection with the sexual life of the child (in the sense in which the word *sexual* is used by Freud), and derive their own pattern largely from it. But there is some difference involved in viewing the death-idea as having a form of its own, as well as a place in the total pattern ; in supposing it to be, as it were, a functional entity or sub-growth, like a limb or a lung, which may become diseased or malformed separately from the rest of the personality, in accordance with separable laws of its own nature, and which if it does this, may then gradually affect the whole in a morbid way.

To speak of an idea as functional is a convenient but somewhat misleading manner of speech. Ideas are not considered, by modern psychologists, to be functioning, motivating entities. It is better to say that when a person's emotional development has reached a certain stage of complexity, then certain aspects of " external reality " lead him to conceive of an idea, such as the idea or the description " dead," " death." The idea is gradually assimilated more and more closely and completely into the memory-patterns (or we may call them complexes, traces, or conditioned-reflex systems) by which each person's impulses are typically directed. During this assimilative process there develops around the concept, as though it were a biological nucleus, a growth or complex of its own, distinguishable from the main system. This sub-complex pursues distinctive processes of development and functions in a distinctive way.

I shall attempt to show that after this particular sub-complex relating to the " dead " idea, has taken distinctive shape, its form and functioning become very important in determining the total emotional and intellectual development of the individual. The functional relationship envisaged between the part and the whole may best be understood by comparing it with processes in other aspects of organic life. Thus, in the constitutional history of England, the development of the courts of Exchequer or of Parliament might be compared with the development of a particular sub-complex in the mental constitution of the individual ; each develops in the closest association with the whole, but in distinctive form, exercising distinctive function, and influencing the development of the whole through its manner of functioning, so deeply that malfunctioning of the minor body may bring about complete disintegration of the major one. Parallels in the development of man's physical body are equally obvious.

In this sense, the idea of death may be said to function. Like Parliament or the eye or the lung, it does not begin functioning in a full and distinctive manner in the earliest periods of the organism's development. The fœtus does not see nor breathe ; nor has the baby made discovery of death. But that does not make the function of seeing or breathing any less important for the man. Eye or lung may function and malfunction distinctively and separably from the rest of the organism, in its physiological aspect ; and in something the same way, the complex which grows up and begins to function around the idea of death may behave and misbehave distinctively and to some extent separably, for the person in his psychological aspect.

To return to the general question : it is of special importance to us at the present time to know what death means to children. But it is really important to know this at all times, and actually we know very little about it, and nothing systematic. Questions about death that are not easily answered and anxieties not easily allayed, occur often in children's nurseries in ordinary times. The grown-up wants to know what the child's questions really mean to the child himself ; what psychological processes lie behind his anxieties ; behind his fears, of the dark or of ghosts, perhaps, or actually of dying. Even the quiet, matter-of-fact questions may be not easy to answer ; and the help and insight that psycho-analysis has given us into the nature and origins of childish anxieties (and that is much) is not always available or sufficient for the parent who is wanting to help an ordinarily-happy child in an immediate crisis of unhappiness.

Yet we must not overrate the importance of understanding the child, as educators have perhaps been inclined to do ever since Rousseau. To understand the child is not the only need, and I would say not the essential need of the adult in his function of rearing the human young. The essential is for the adult to provide something from his own resources ; to transmit sustenance, whether in the form of food, knowledge, wisdom, or cultural tradition. To understand the child is to be aware (consciously or unconsciously) how much the sustenance needs to be predigested. But whether the milk is suitable for the infant is, however important, secondary to ensuring that the infant is fed at all.

Essentially, what the adult gives the child, in the way of suggestion or response, in connection with this subject of death, will depend very largely upon his own resources, his own attitude, and the social culture and traditions to which he has reacted. If he is deeply imbued with a culture that is rich and well adapted to individual and social needs he may, by handing it on to the child, help to build in him a mental structure strong to withstand the inevitable strains of life. If he fails to do this, it may be because of the poverty of the culture, or its inflexibility relative to a changing social environment, or the fact that he has not deeply experienced a single cultural influence, but, under influences very complex or conflicting, has himself found no stable or stabilizing attitude to life or death. And to-day this may easily happen, for our European culture is not poor nor inflexible, but its richness and flexibility are gained at the cost of including much that seems quite irreconcilable, and the individual, offered so many and such various patterns for life, may attempt to accommodate himself to many, and fully accept none.

The social organization of human reactions to the fact

and the thought of death has always been a function of *religion.* Religion socializes individual attitudes to death. It provides a definite pattern for them, and makes that pattern to be considered sane. It is the name given to traditionally tested ways of mental acceptance of death.

For the idea is not easy to accept. The fact is deeply written into the records of mankind. It can be seen to underlie the most diverse beliefs and social reactions. Some primitive peoples deny the necessity of physical death, and attribute all death to individual accidents. Others who do not deny that it is inevitable, react to it with elaborate funeral ceremonies, sometimes of a very violent nature, in which customary restraints on behaviour and particularly on sexual intercourse are loosened, and obscenities and jests are encouraged which mock dying and the dead. Many people, including many of the most highly civilized, deny the completeness of death for the individual, and in their creeds and rituals express a belief in personal immortality either of the soul, or of soul and body, too. Socrates refused to grieve at his own death, saying it would set his soul free, but he could not keep his friends from weeping.

The idea is not easy to accept. Many of the greatest thinkers have not accepted the idea that when the body decays there is also a complete dissolution of the personality. Yet others have (consciously, at least) accepted that idea. In the face of death, religion may still perform functions for those who do not believe in personal immortality. European religion has for so many centuries been bound up with beliefs in personal immortality that this is seldom realized. There was a period, in ancient Rome, when the living said farewell for ever to the dead, as Catullus did to his brother ; and yet Catullus journeyed far over land and sea to pay to his brother the last funeral tributes. Religion still offers its rites and consolations even when farewell is felt as final, and if those rites bring death into a grand and positive relation with life, they must have social value.

What death means and may mean to children cannot really be considered fully, apart from what it means to the adults who rear the children and to the whole society and tradition in contact with which they live. But the larger questions may be considered for a time as the background, and attention may be focused meanwhile on the children's actual, momentary reactions to this subject, when those reactions are, as it were, isolated and put under the microscope. In the last chapter I shall try to relate the findings to some of these larger aspects of the question which, all through, will be visibly looming in the background. Also I shall try to show what the observations imply in terms of practical life, for those concerned with the day-to-day handling of young children, and further, what contribution they may offer to the science of child psychology.

CHAPTER II

THREE methods were used to collect material directly from children about their own ways of thinking about death. These were, firstly, records taken at home by parents; secondly, a Story-Completion Test; thirdly, the giving of a well-known intelligence test, with certain additions in what was given and in the keeping of special records of some of the responses.

CONSIDERATIONS GOVERNING THE CHOICE OF METHODS

The aim was to obtain material over a wide age-range, and at different levels of thought. The word " levels " is here used metaphorically in the usual way, the " deeper " mental processes being considered as the unconscious, autistic or dream-like modes of mental functioning, and the " upper " being distinguished by having more distinct aims, of which the thinker is aware all through the process itself; this is called conscious or directive thought.

The choice of method was determined mainly by three considerations. (1) There should be a large proportion of relevant material, in proportion to the total gathered. (2) It should be possible to treat it objectively (so that, for instance, it would not be possible for behaviour to be classed as illuminating by one observer, of which another observer might say : " The child had no idea of death when he did that, any more than a dog when he kills a fly on the window-pane ") ; to record it objectively in manageable compass ;

8

to classify results, and to arrange for some degree of quantitative treatment of them. (3) Lastly, it was very important to find a way to circumvent happily the reserves and resistances which prevent access to others' minds, falsify what is given, or limit the levels of thought from which it is drawn.

The first consideration led to the rejection of several methods which have already, in other researches with somewhat different aims, brought in material relevant to this research.[1]

Because of the second consideration, and especially the need to avoid subjective interpretations as much as possible, and to collect material which could be easily presented, verbal material has been relied upon more than any other kind. This is not from an opinion that the individual significance of ideas is solely or most truthfully expressed in words. It is because of the difficulty of determining objectively what ideas are being expressed by behaviour which is not verbal, nor accompanied by words, nor subsequently referred to in words. General behaviour, such as play, or specific behaviour, such as closing the eyes or sucking a finger when speaking about death, have not passed unnoticed, but they have only been used as direct material when there was also some verbal reference to the idea.

As regards circumvention of resistance, it has been taken as axiomatic that a stranger does not obtain reliable responses from a child about his most recently achieved integrations of conscious thought, and an intimate does not obtain reliable responses to questions that touch upon feelings and fantasies, unless the child is provided with a substitute for the defences that normally guard the core of personality. Resistance is a protective shell which fulfils a necessary

[1] See F. C. Bartlett's study, *Remembering*, and R. Griffiths' *Study of Imagination in Early Childhood*, for examples of other techniques which might profitably be employed.

function. Direct attack upon it is an unwarrantable aggression and tactically ineffective. The child so approached may close up, like a sea-anemone or a wood-louse ; or he may display himself, like the lapwing when her nest is approached, who, of course, does not display her nest but cleverly conceals it. The child who does not show the resistance normal to its age and social environment is not a normal child. There are instances in these records of responses from such children (see Edna K., p. 37). A method of direct personal approach overweights the importance of this type.

Circumvention of resistance, however, can be a friendly act. It may actually strengthen the defences, by recognizing their existence and yet at the same time offering social contact.

On these grounds, therefore, direct questions with personal implications were ruled out from the routine procedure. For the same reason the responses obtained in other researches based on a routine of direct questions have not been used.

Two main lines of approach remained. The first : to record children's spontaneous remarks, questions, and behaviour. This (the recording of questions) was the method suggested by Professor Piaget (in a personal interview). His own use of it, as described in his work, *The Language and Thought of the Child*, was scientifically systematized, and produced some very interesting material relevant to the subject of the conception of death in children. In that form, however, it could not be used for this research ; to apply it to a sufficient number of children for a sufficient time, a large team of workers would be needed. For this research it has also specific disadvantages. Children may tend to ask different types of question at different times of day, or of certain people. Questions about death may be reserved for the mother at bed-time. In my experience, cosmic speculations usually occur during family meals, and hypotheses about the ultimate destiny of the body, during the bath. Consequently the method of systematically recording spontaneous questions and remarks does not give a proportioned or complete picture of the content of childish thought, when its application is limited to certain times of day or certain observers. The difficulty is increased with certain subjects of thought, such as death. But if the application is less restricted, much of the scientific value of the method is lost.

In the Home Records an attempt has been made to use this method in the simpler, wider way, and yet with a minimum of error.

Constant use has also been made of published observations made in this way by eminent psychologists ; more particularly of the work of Sully, the Sterns, Rasmussen, the Katz's, and Dr. Susan Isaacs.

The second line of approach is through the provision of other defences to take the place of verbal resistance. *Projection* offers such an alternative. This process can take various forms. It always involves a partial detachment or dissociation of the personality. The small infant expresses himself in play : the soldier whom he makes shoot the doll is, and at the same time is not, the child himself. Such simple substitution of another material figure for the self is one of the early types of projection. Still at a comparatively early stage of development, an ideal image may take the place of the material figure. *A little boy once upon a time* fulfils the function of the toy soldier, and a witch that of the doll. Provided with such a screen for simple projection, the child will express himself in fantasies that involve his affective life, and often relieve and enjoy himself through the act of expression. These were the main psychological considerations leading to the choice of the Story-Completion Test.

Using the doll or the witch, the soldier or the story-hero, the child can dissociate from the perceiving self those affective activities which preoccupy his mind. When projection and temporary dissociation take this form, it is the affective complex which is externalized from the individual.

The same mechanism may be used in the opposite way. In place of the affective complex, we have the perceptual complex which is sometimes called an object or thing. The individual now keeps as his own all affect—feeling, suffering, loving—while he projects from himself the *thing*, object, or perceptual complex, and views it as independent of himself. Of course the object perceived is not in fact independent ; there may be external reality, but it is not synonymous with things perceived. But this projection of the perceptual complex (which is simply the psychological basis of science, and its fundamental technique) provides us with another method of circumventing resistances ; a very simple one, namely, the suggestion of an objective or scientific attitude. By voice and manner it is suggested to the child that all personal feelings have been set aside : perceptual material or ideas (that is to say, objects or verbal problems) are presented to be studied " for their own sake," and it is taken for granted that affect (feeling) is not involved.

A psycho-analytical interpretation of this technique is, that we suggest to the subject to use in his defence a type of reaction which (carried to extremes of manner or habit) is obsessional-neurotic, rather than one which (carried to extremes) is hysterical. The hysteric mechanism of defence is to fall silent—to find a blank in the mind—when repressed material comes into the associative train, whereas the obsessional-neurotic " does not fall silent ; he speaks, even when in a state of resistance. But he severs the links between his associations and isolates ideas from affects when he is speaking " (20.*b*.i).

It will be noted later (p. 81) that this technique was unsuccessful with 6 out of 91 children studied : the impulse towards the hysterical (verbal inhibition) reaction was too strong in them for this counter-suggestion towards another type of defence to take effect. Milder hysterical types some-times revealed themselves through physical action accom-panying the response ; shutting of eyes or sucking of fingers was the commonest form of this type of reaction.

Some framework cutting off the period of objective dissociation from the more complete ordinary life is as necessary as the framework of the Story-Completion Test for separating the period of dissociated affect. This second framework was found in the Binet Intelligence Tests, used in the revision and with the additions described below. The essential element for this purpose is the correct, standardized manner of administering the tests—friendly but objective—rather than their content. Actually, much of the content also is relevant to the purpose. Anything more that is wanted can be easily added, whereas without the framework of the test-situation, the same questions would appear as an incredibly clumsy attempt to penetrate the most private sanctums of thought and emotion.

THE METHODS AND SUBJECTS

1.—*Home Records*

(*a*) Methods

In five families including the writer's own, parents consented to take records of their children's questions, remarks, or responses on the subject of death.

Each family was given a notebook for the records, in which were entered the names and birth-dates of the children, a calendar, and certain detailed instructions to ensure the recording of the date, time of day, activity in progress, the interval (if any) ensuing between the incident and the recording of it, the persons present, and the accom-panying and subsequent behaviour of the child.

Each parent who consented to keep such a record was personally interviewed before the notebook entries began. It was made clear that every reference to the subject of research would be considered of value, and that delay in entering an account of an incident reduced the value of the record.

The great majority of the entries were made by the mothers of the children. A small number were made by fathers. One was reported to the mother by the nurse, and entered immediately by the mother.

A considerable number of the entries were made simultaneously in shorthand. Some were made a considerable time after the incident recorded. The latter have not been invariably rejected, but when used, note has been made of the delay, and the admission of these records has been only for the purpose of illuminating other incidents reported with greater exactitude.

(*b*) The Subjects used for Home Records

These records refer to eleven children, living in five different families. In two of these families there was also a younger brother who had not yet learned to speak. None of the subjects were only children. None of them had had experience of the death of siblings or parents.

The pseudonyms chosen for the children show the sibling relationships, but not the cousin relationships. Mr. Anson is brother to Mrs. Holme ; Mrs. Anson is sister to Mr. Clement.

The children, in age order

1. Catherine Holland
2. Margaret Sage
3. Benedict Clement (Ben)
4. Susanna Holland
5. Judith Anson
6. Jeremy Sage
7. Richard Clement
8. Francis Holland
9. Stephen Holme
10. Timothy Anson
11. Edward Holme

and younger brothers :
> Anthony Sage
> John Holland.

All the children were acquainted with each other, except that Stephen and Edward Holme, who lived some miles away, were unacquainted with the Hollands and the Sages. All the other children attended the same school (a private preparatory school) at some time during the taking of the records ; Ben, however, had left, to attend another private school (for boys only) before Richard, Francis or Timothy came.

Intelligence. The head teacher of this school which most of the children at some time attended, did not wish parents to have information of the intelligence test results of their own or others' children. This decision obviously had to be respected. With four of the children, however, the ban did not apply. These children, tested on Stanford-Binet Scale, scored I.Q.'s ranging from 132 to 172. This result was obtained by a well qualified and experienced psychologist on the earlier Stanford-Binet revision when the child was aged 6. General observation of the children suggests that no child would be badly left out if this range were given for the total number of the children.

The *socio-economic status* of the five families was roughly similar at the time the study was made. Seven of the parents were University graduates (representing Oxford, Cambridge, London and Edinburgh). None were school teachers, medical practitioners, clergy, or (except the writer) students of psychology.

Of the *religious upbringing* of the children little can be said. When at school they all heard readings from the Bible, and were told, or acted, gospel stories at Christmas time. Among the ten parents, four had been brought up in families of Unitarian tradition (Protestant Nonconformist), three in the Church of England. One was Jewish, but did not practise traditional observances. Of two, information on the matter of religious belief or upbringing is lacking. The prevalence of agnosticism is not known ; nor can the early influence of nurses and domestic servants be estimated, though reference to such influences appears in the records.

2.—*The Story-Completion Test*

This test, devised at the Institut Jean-Jacques Rousseau of Geneva and published in the Geneva *Archives de Psychologie* (71), consists of a series of brief story-openings which the child is invited to complete, verbally. It is not a mental test in the usual sense ; that is to say, it is not intended to give a quantitative measure of a mental ability, but it is planned as a clinical technique, to discover as rapidly and surely as possible the pattern and the tangles of the child's emotional life.

These story-openings make no reference to death. But when the test was first used, in Geneva, it was found that the subject appeared constantly in the children's responses (their completions of the stories), and actually 66 per cent of the children brought it in.

It therefore seemed to offer a magnificent instrument for the special purpose of discovering how children think about death in their fantasies, and for this purpose it was translated, and tried on children in an English Child Guidance Clinic (where it has remained in general use). In the English translation certain minor changes were made from the Geneva version, and as finally used it stood as follows :

STORY-COMPLETION TEST

1. A boy (little boy, girl, little girl) went to school ; when play-time came, he didn't play with the others, but stayed all alone in a corner. Why ?

2. A boy was quarrelling with his brother (sister), and their mother came up to them, and then . . . what happened ?

3. A boy was having dinner with his mother and father. The father got very angry, because . . . Why ?

4. One day the father and mother were annoyed with each other, and they quarrelled, and the reason was . . . ?

5. One Sunday the boy (or, they all) went out for the day with his (their) father and mother ; when they came home in the evening the mother was very sad. Why ?

6. The boy had a friend he liked very much ; one day this friend came to him and said, " You come with me and I'll tell you a secret, and show you something, but you mustn't tell anyone about it ! " What did he show him ; what did he tell him ?

7a. When the boy went to bed at night-time, what did he think about ?

7b. One night he cried when he went to bed ; he was very unhappy. Why was that ?

8a. Then he went to sleep, and what did he dream about ?

8b. He woke up again, in the middle of the night, and was very frightened. Why ?

9. Then he went to sleep again, and this time he had a lovely dream : a fairy appeared to him and said, " I can make anything you wish come true ; tell me what you want, and then I will touch you with my magic wand and your wish will come true. You can have three wishes." What did he ask for ?

10. Then the fairy said, " You are growing into a big boy ; do you want to be big and grown-up, or would you like to stay a child for a long time, perhaps for always ? " The boy said . . . What did he say ?

11. Then the fairy gave him £100,000 to spend. What did he do with it ?

---

12. Shall we change round : you tell some stories and ask me about what happened then or why, and I have to tell the rest ?

ADMINISTRATION OF THE STORY-COMPLETION TEST

Although the test was used as an experimental technique, there was no insistence on identity of environmental

c

conditions for its administration. In three different London school buildings, and the garden of a rural school, in two clinics, in a suburban garden of the child's own home, in the study of a country vicarage and in that garden—the only environmental conditions which were considered essential in every situation were privacy, seats, a table, and writing materials.

All answers were recorded word for word, if necessary in shorthand. Subjects were never asked to speak more slowly or distinctly, or to repeat statements. Longhand writing was used for recording when possible, because of the difficulty of accurately rendering and deciphering in shorthand the many dialect and childish variants of English presented. Much is lost inevitably in the transcription from tongue to type which is significant to the sociologist and psychologist ; the loss is much increased when the transcription is a double process, and neither script accurately phonetic. But so that every word should be transcribed, many responses, particularly from the more voluble of the older children, had to be recorded in shorthand. In the opinion of the experi-menter, the Story-Completion Test demands shorthand for trustworthy recording of responses.

Before the story-telling began, the experimenter had a little talk with the child, sometimes on the way from the playground or classroom to the story-telling room. During this time the child was asked about his family—whether he had any brothers or sisters, older or younger, and so on. No other particulars were asked, though they were sometimes spontaneously given.

The Geneva devisers of the Story-Completion Test insist that it is not a test in the usual sense, but a clinical technique ; successful use of it, from the clinical point of view, does not depend on standardization of procedure, but on adaptation to each individual child, so as to get a similar and full degree of confidence. In this research, however, the test was administered in a comparatively standardized way. No additional stories were added, even if emotional complexities remained unresolved. The child was not pressed to develop his fantasies to the full. Follow-up queries were only put to him when he was unusually brief, or obviously showed a desire for such encouragement. The aim in this case (unlike that of the clinicians) was not so much to plumb the depths of each individual child's affective life, as to observe the variations of fantasy which arose in consciousness as an immediate response to fantasy suggestions. If a child were unusually garrulous, following-up questions were reduced or avoided ; if he were normally responsive, then a point of interest left outstanding in the completion might elicit " And then ? " or " Did he often. . . ? " or some such encouragement to enlarge the matter. A child whose resistances inhibited speech would be encouraged in this way if the desire to confide seemed to be impelling him beyond his powers of expression. Children approaching the age for taking scholarship examinations occasionally became much freer in fantasy-expression when reminded that the test had nothing to do with school work.

In some cases story 4 was omitted ; that is, when the family was personally known to the experimenter, or when the child had lost one or both parents and was himself still young, so that the inapplicability of the story to himself might cause a break in the identification process.

IDENTIFICATION

The value of the Story-Completion Test for the present purpose depends on the child's identification of himself with the " hero " of the stories. He has not himself selected the screen for projection, as he does in his own spontaneous fantasy. Identification will depend on the story evoking a situation, a mental attitude, that he feels himself to have experienced. If that does occur, then, as Mdlle. Thomas writes :

" le complexe énoncé dans l'histoire, correspondant à un complexe analogue chez l'enfant, déclenchera une réaction affective ; tout comme en acoustique un corps en vibration déclenche la vibration d'un autre corps du même diapason " (71.i).

The fact that the child identifies himself with the " hero " of some or all the stories is shown in different ways. With not one of the subjects was the impression given that identification failed to occur at some stage. Usually it was apparent throughout the test. Sometimes the identification was only verified in the light of further information about the child's actual or fantasy experience.

Identification may be shown by the child stating the parallelism of his story-response and his own life ; or by a direct response in terms of his own life; or by resistance. To give examples of these three types of response :

Ian S.,[1]   8 : 3
7a. I *am* caught in a trap now ! He'd better go to sleep. I generally go to sleep. Everybody does, don't they ?

8a. Dreamt about 'is sweet'eart—some people do, don't they ? (Q. What's his sweetheart's name ?) Pamela X. (Q. Is she nice ?) Not 'alf ! (Q. How old is she ?) Eight and three-quarters. She lives down at the bottom of the road.

10. " No," the boy would say, " I'd rather grow up to be a man." *I* would. I'd be a bus driver. My friend, Uncle Jim, is.

Another example of parallelism is that of Willie K., 6 : 7 :

8b. (The boy was frightened in the night.) Because it was so dark, and he thought it was someone in 'is 'ouse—a ghost or somebody—or a burglar. I suppose 'e 'eard a

---

[1] The initial used for the child's second name indicates his intelligence level, M. being Average, A. Maximum and Z. Minimum. Ian S. is thus a dull boy.

sound—a noise—might've been a ghost of somebody.
That's what I'm frightened of . . . because I went to the
pictures and I saw a man with eyes as big as that ! . . . 'E
killed 'isself—'e dressed some man up as a ghost, and 'e
killed 'im. I think about bears with 'im and all. (Q. Were
there bears in the picture ?) No, but I just think about them,
too. I think of them under the bed. Then I run downstairs
to my mum. . . .

We may believe, though we cannot prove, that Bill H.,
7 : o, was identifying himself with the " hero " when he
answered story 7*b* (why the boy was unhappy when he went
to bed) :

" Because he was cold. E' 'ad no clothes on 'im much."

And it is difficult to resist the conclusion, when the same boy
answers story 9 (the three wishes) as follows :

" 'E wished 'e could be a good boy for always. 'E wished
'e could grow up as a man and 'ave a motor-car, and 'ave
good jobs. And the other one was, to keep 'is 'andkerchief
and not always 'ave a dirty nose in school."

Bill is very pale and extremely thin. His elder brother
and younger sister have both died of diphtheria.
This last response of Bill's is identification in direct terms
of his own life. It is his real life. We also get identification
of the " hero " with the child's fantasy life. Josephine Q., a
clinic case aged 9 : 1, could think of no response for her
heroine, to the offer of three wishes, but that " Nothing
would do her harm." Another clinical case, Norman D.,
aged 6 : o, stated the parallelism between his completion
of story 8*a* and his habitual fantasies :

(The boy dreamed) he was in a lavatory doing poops and
someone came along and pulled the chain, and when the
water went down, he went down too. I dreamed that last

night. I've dreamt it twenty-four times. The night before, that was the twenty-third time.

Resistance is often shown by non-verbal behaviour. At certain story-openings the child makes no reply at all, or there is an exceptionally long pause. One little girl, Margaret E., aged 7 : 8, would open her mouth to speak and then shut and purse it up, again and again, during such silences. Ian S.'s answers (p. 20), give an example of resistance expressed in words. Lily O., aged 10 : 5, who had to be reassured that the test had nothing to do with school-work before her manner showed any freedom, answered story 9 (the three wishes) as follows :

" That she would not have any more—No ! That she would not have any more funny dreams—you know—That she could have all the money she wanted—and all the nice clothes she wanted."

Two of the nine-year-old boys, Desmond I. and Dennis Q., answered each story readily until it came to 8b (why the boy was frightened in the night), but at this were involved in resistances. Desmond, after long silence, said, " Don't know " ; Dennis repeated " Frightened, frightened . . ." to himself, and then fitted the responses into his fantasy-series of cruel bird's-nesting, and the consequent sense of guilt. Henry F., aged 6 : 2, opens his series of responses with an obvious resistance : the boy did not play with the others " 'Cos 'e was n . . . cold."

COMPLICATIONS OF IDENTIFICATION

The identification with the fantasy-self sometimes cuts across the identification with the self of real experience. In consequence of this, although there may in every case be identification, one cannot conclude that the child's own experience is being drawn upon for the description of what happens to the "hero," or that the "hero's" wishes are the real (as distinct from the fantasy) wishes of the child. For example, a London school-boy aged 7 : 3, Freddy P., when asked how he would spend £100,000, answers "Buy an 'orse." His fantasy-wish for his grown-up occupation is to be a soldier and shoot ; in his own person he decides to be an engine-driver. Where does the horse come in ? After school, Freddy says, he is going to play a game of "swanking," as a cowboy ; he uses the other boys as his horses, choosing those that do not get out of breath, and whips them with a bit of string if they don't go fast enough ; this is evidently the central interest of his life at present. In this game he has his regular name as the cowboy slave-driver ; the whole fantasy is excellently organized, and fully carried out in objective material. Freddy has projected this half-fantasy, half-reality aspect of his personality into the story and the completion of it.

Another influence tends to draw the projection away from simple reflection of "real" aspects of experience ; this influence is similar to the process of *closure* observed in perceptual experience. Just as certain shapes and patterns are automatically registered by the mind as conforming to a conventional type which they actually only partially resemble, so some fantasy-situations have conventionally-correct resolutions, which the child will occasionally supply, rather than resolve them in a way based on individual experience that is felt to be more peculiar. The individual way would be like ending a fairy-story, not with the hero and heroine marrying and living happily ever after, but by their breaking their betrothal, just because one's aunt happened to have done that. The generalization or closure process is most likely to occur in response to the earlier stories, when fantasy has not yet become confidently individual. It is, however, the exception rather than the rule, even with the first response. "Because he was naughty" is the conventional response to story 1 ; it is probably the response against which Henry F. exerted resistance (see p. 22).

In interpreting each individual case, therefore, it is necessary to know what is the beaten-track of fantasy, and allow for a constant tendency to revert to it.

3.—*The Intelligence Test with Additions*

(*a*) The Tests

The first consideration in the choice of an Intelligence Test was to provide a setting for the objective insulation of questions charged with strong emotional tone. The second consideration was to obtain a rating of the children's intellectual development on a well-standardized scale.

No test could fulfil the first requirement unless it contained a good deal of verbal material. The second requirement was not so much a fine accuracy in measurement of g (that is, the general factor in mental ability which, according to Spearman, is measured by validly constructed intelligence tests), as the ranking of all the children on an Intelligence Scale in common use and esteem.

The revised Binet scale was chosen as best fulfilling this requirement as well as the need for verbal material. In every case at least one other well-standardized test was given, based on non-verbal processes, but only the results of the Binet tests have been used for the final assessment of the child's mental age and intelligence.[1]   The form of Binet

---

[1] *Assessment of the child's mental age and intelligence.*
The results of testing intelligence are conventionally scored in two different ways. In both, the child's total score is reckoned as a " mental age," and this score is then divided by the actual (chronological) age. The tests are framed so as to make the " mental age " and the chronological age equal for children of average (mean) intelligence.
The ratio of mental : chronological age can then be expressed either as an I.Q. or in standard score. For an I.Q. score, the ratio is multiplied by 100, so as to avoid fractions. A score of exactly 100 therefore indicates that a child is of exactly average intelligence. For a standard score, the average ratio is taken as 0, and the unit of reckoning is the standard deviation of a normal distribution, with a possible range from —5

scale chosen was Form L of Stanford-Binet revision, 1937, made in America by Terman and Merrill and modified for English use in the simultaneous English publication (70). Many of the children were tested on the abbreviated scale (but without omitting specially relevant tests).

Apart from its claim as the scale in most common use for intelligence-testing in this country, the Binet tests had the special advantage of bringing in the subject of death to an unusual and rather surprising extent. In Binet's original work this feature was still more marked. Early users of the scale encountered a girl cut up into eighteen pieces, who was supposed to have chosen this method of killing herself; and there were other items not much less gruesome. The Revised Version has cut out some of these sensational features, whether after studying their psychological effects upon the children or simply because of a general change in adult attitude remains unknown. While this was unknown, it was thought better to err on the side of prudence, and use that version of the Binet tests which was most up to date. In the revised version there still remains much material

(complete idiocy) to +5 (" genius "), and a practical range from —3 (low-grade mental defect) to +3 (good university standard).

In actual practice, all scores in the present work have been found as I.Q.'s (with the help of the tables at the end of Terman and Merrill's *Measuring Intelligence*), and if it was desired to reckon also the standard score, they were then converted, on the basis of a standard deviation of 16 or 17 I.Q. points to the unit.

This gives a range of 20 to 180 I.Q. as equivalent to a range of ±5 in standard scores. Normally, 68 per cent of a population will make scores ranging between 84 and 116 I.Q. (or, ±1 standard score). An I.Q. of 70 is commonly taken as the frontier between mental deficiency and " normal " intelligence; it is approximately equivalent to —2 standard score.

To give the term *mental age* to a score obtained by " intelligence " testing is to assume that the mind matures simultaneously in every functional aspect. This assumption is probably unsound. The term *intelligence-age*, as applied to intelligence-testing, would be preferable; but the usual practice has nevertheless been followed here.

which is relevant to researches on children's ideas of death. These relevant items are tabulated below :

" VERBAL ABSURDITIES " TESTS

The procedure for administering these tests is given as follows : " Read each statement and, after each one, ask, ' What is foolish about that ? ' If the response is ambiguous without further explanation ask, ' Why is that (it) foolish ? ' " (70.i). (English testers commonly substitute " silly " for foolish.)

Year.   *Test No.*

VIII.   3c.   " I read in the paper that the police fired two shots at a man. The first shot killed him, but the second did not hurt him much."

IX.   2d.   " In an old graveyard in Spain they have
(or   discovered a small skull which they believe to
XII.   2d.)   be that of Christopher Columbus when he was about ten years old."

XI.   2a.   " The judge said to the prisoner, ' You are to be hanged, and I hope it will be a warning to you.' "

XI.   2b.   " A well-known railway had its last accident five years ago, and since that time only one person has been killed on it in an accident."

" PROBLEMS OF FACT "

The procedure is for the tester to say, " Listen," and then to recite the problem. Further procedure in the event of certain types of response is added for each problem (70.ii)

Year   *Test No.*

XIII.   4a.   " A man who was walking in the woods near a town stopped suddenly, very much frightened, and then ran to the nearest policeman, saying that he had just seen hanging from the limb of a tree a . . . a what ? " (If the reply is " man," say, " Tell me what you mean ; explain it.")

4*b*.   " My neighbour has been having queer
visitors. First a doctor came to his house, then
a lawyer, then a minister (preacher, priest, or
rabbi). What do you think happened there ? "
(If the response is " a death," etc., check by
asking what the lawyer came for.)

In administering these tests the following changes were
made :

(*a*) IX.2*d*. A hero more familiar to the English child was
substituted for Christopher Columbus (usually William the
Conqueror) and the reference to Spain was omitted.

(*b*) XIII.4*a*. The word *branch* was substituted for the word
limb.

(*c*) XIII.4*b*. The word *clergyman* was allowed as a
substitute for *minister*.

An addition was also made to the scale by adding the
word " dead " to the Vocabulary List between the words
" puddle " and " tap " (numbers 4 and 5 on the list).
Another verbal adjective, " sold," was also added at some
earlier point in the list. This was done so as to accustom
the child to the different grammatical type of the word
" dead " from the other words in the list, which are nouns
up till No. 18 (" priceless ") ; and also to provide a comparison in respect of the delay of response attributable to
different grammatical type. The measure is, of course, very
rough, for delay due to such a cause may be expected to
diminish with the second word of the same grammatical
category. The procedure was planned rather as a safeguard
against attributing any observed delay in the " dead "
response, to the idea in the word and the inhibition of
affective complexes alone, since there were other factors
involved, such as this one of grammar.

Reaction-times were not recorded. Responses to all
questions involving the idea of death were taken down word
for word.

The children tested numbered 117 in all. Seventy-five of
these were given both the Story-Completion and the
Intelligence Tests.   Twenty-three were not given the
additions to the Intelligence Test ; fifteen were not given the
Story-Completion. The omission of the Intelligence Test
was because the children had been recently tested by other
people on the same scale. This happened mainly with
clinical cases. The omission of the Story-Completion Tests
was due to privacy being unobtainable, or to the child's
mental age being too low : a child of mental age under 5 : 0
may be unable to respond to it.

How were the children selected ? One wants, of course,
a representative sample of the whole population, for such a
theme as this. Theoretically, a representative sample is
obtained by random selection, and the probability of its
reactions being really representative is proportional to the
size of the sample. But, of course, we cannot make a random
selection from our population while it is riddled with
segregations necessary to its functioning. Thus, if we want
our sample of children to show a normal distribution of
intelligence, and to be largely drawn from urban areas, we
shall have to go purposely to Special Schools for Mental
Defectives to secure responses from some children with
intelligence below 70 I.Q.

So we have to decide how many of the deficient children
to take, and we may determine our figure on the basis of
making the distribution in our sample parallel with normal
distribution, or we may make some other decision. What
we cannot do, with regard to intelligence or other qualities,
is to obtain by random methods a sample which will have
the qualities of a random sample in the statistical sense of
the term, and so be truly representative of children (or even
English children) in general.

Since the distribution of our sample will therefore partly depend on our own prior decisions and assumptions it proves little in itself, and a good case can be made for not attempting to reproduce normal distribution in miniature but in over-weighting the extremes. Otherwise, in a sample of only 100 children, we might reasonably have no extreme cases, and certainly no possibility, if such did appear, of knowing whether their reactions were characteristic of the extreme, or purely individual.

The aim, in this study, was therefore to keep to a normal distribution only in so far as that resulted from the random selection of the majority of the children from among those being educated in ordinary English council schools before the outbreak of war. Overweighting of the extremes of deficiency and intelligence was permitted, so that there might be some comparison of examples at those extremes. But the overweighting was limited, with the intention of keeping the centre of interest and attention focused on the child of average ability.

The majority of the children (65) were drawn from two council schools in south-east London. The rest of the " normal " children were three boys and two girls tested privately, and ten children living in a small country village in Leicestershire.

Eleven cases were tested in Special (non-residential) Schools for Mental Defectives. Twenty-six cases were seen at Child Guidance Clinics, which between them served a wide area in and around London.[1]

It might seem an easy matter to study an equal number of boys and girls, and so imitate the normal distribution of sex at school. Actually it was not so simple. The number of boys referred to clinics is greater than the number of girls,

[1] One boy in a Special School was found to have an intelligence score above deficiency level (a result confirmed by the headmaster and the medical officer). One girl in an ordinary school scored below the deficiency level. The history, afterwards reported, strongly suggested that the child's intelligence had deteriorated owing to epilepsy.

and this proportion was reflected in the number of clinical cases studied. Socially-determined sex differences operated to produce the same effect in the small rural group. The local schools were not in session, but the ground had been prepared for friendly contacts. The children were invited to come to the house to be tested, other attractions being placed in the forefront of the programme. The village was very scattered, and there was no convenient means of public transport to the house. The consequence was that six boys, all of whom had bicycles, availed themselves of the invitation, and indeed came with cumulative frequency, but no girls (the girls had not bicycles). The local infants' school opened again as the visit came to a close ; out of ten children only two were girls, who were immediately tested, and also two more boys.

To equalize the numbers of "normal" boys and girls studied, the number of London girls taken was rather more than the number of boys, as will be seen from the table below. Apart from clinic cases there were 40 boys and 40 girls scoring above the defective-intelligence level, because of the non-defective boy in the Special School and the defective girl in the ordinary school. This fact does not show in the table, but it explains why the number of ordinary school boys and girls are unequal (boys 39, girls 41).

TABLE I

Showing the Distribution of the Children Tested, according to Sex and Institution

Sex	Ordinary Schools			Special Schools (M.D.)	Referred to Clinics	TOTAL
	L.C.C.	Private	Rural			
Boys ..	28	3	8	8	17	64
Girls ..	37	2	2	3	9	53
TOTAL	65	5	10	11	26	117

CHAPTER III

DEATH IN CHILDREN'S FANTASIES

FREUD has said that to the child death means little more than departure or disappearance, and that it is represented in dreams by going on a journey. He has also said that there is no unconscious correlative to be found for the conscious concept of death (21.c).

The concepts which psycho-analysis finds in the unconscious mind can be interpreted in this way, on general principles, but they may also have to be interpreted differently in individual cases. Sometimes going a journey may not imply a thought of death ; at other times a thought of death may be represented in a different way. And on the other hand, when we, adults or children, deal explicitly with the subject of death, psycho-analysis shows us that that idea may stand for some quite other concept in the unconscious mind.

Fantasies expressed in words—fairy-stories and the like— occupy a realm halfway between fully conscious or directive thought and the unconscious thought of dreams. If we are to try to find out how the child's mind is working when he uses words referring unambiguously to death in his fantasies, we must consider first this problem of what a word represents.

The word is a symbol for the whole meaning ; and the meaning is a mental integration of a multitude of perceptions (directly experienced or else suggested) which, thanks to immediate need or to social tradition, are in practice dealt with together. This complex whole which is the meaning of a word (or may sometimes be called the idea behind the word) may be likened in metaphor to a multiple-stringed musical instrument (say, a violin), which may be set vibrating all over, or in part only, with an immense variety of response. The analogy would be closer if violins could grow.

A concept is the effect of an actual stimulation of this instrument. Thus one kind of stimulation produces an unconscious concept and another a conscious concept, but a unitary meaning or idea underlies both.

We cannot strictly keep to this usage of words and may sometimes use the word concept for the whole complex, or alternatively narrow down *concept* or *idea* to mean the symbol by which the concept is represented.

Unconscious concepts are said to inhabit the Id, the imagined abode of the most fundamental psychic impulses. At the Id's lower threshold, bodily and mental impulses join hands in some mysterious way ; at its upper threshold, impulses may become conscious. The impulses in the Id give rise to concepts which, if brought to consciousness, appear most easily in the form of pictures, visual images. In their simplest form these picture-symbols are commonly based on some analogy of perceptual resemblance or difference ; a ring, for instance, represents a body-orifice, an apple the mother's breast, and so on.

Picture-symbols can represent an idea as it was formed before language was learned. But words, once learned, may symbolize a whole conceptual complex, including the simplest, earliest form of it. Through word-stimulation the whole complex may be set vibrating in all or any of its parts.

Consequently, all behavioural expansions which the person explicitly connects with the word give the observer some light on its meaning for him. A behavioural expansion may be, for instance, the verbal response to a request for a definition of " dead," or a purely motor activity which is in any way connected with the word. One child, aged five, when asked the meaning of " dead," acted the collision of two toy cars with the clearest intention of expressing that meaning ; this was his behavioural expansion of it. A middle-aged man attending a department of psychological medicine for a neurosis which took the form of a fear of death, and prevented him from carrying out his work as an engine-driver, was observed to shut his eyes when he spoke of death : a reaction sometimes seen in younger people who are apparently in normal health. Such reactions help to show what death means to them.

In this attempt to find out what death means, and how children discover it, the *word* has been used throughout as the guiding line, and we have never let it go, not because it was supposed that meanings (conceptual complexes) were only or even best expressed in words, but because through the word we can eventually reach to the furthest boundaries of the complex, and because, since the whole mind is ultimately connected, once we let go of the word, we may without knowing it pass beyond a rightful frontier.

Sometimes very early impulses of the child are referred to as " death-wishes " : these are feelings of fury, violent aggressiveness and cannibalism against those persons or objects which frustrate the infant. Such feelings, in later manifestations, a child may associate with the conscious concept of death. But when the feelings first occur he cannot do so, for the distinctive complex which the word refers to has not yet developed. He has no more discovered death than the fœtus has discovered light. The association of these feelings with the idea of death is made by the analyst or the observer, not by the child. Indeed, the observer might go further if he wished, and speak of pre-natal death-wishes, when the baby and mother compete for nourishment (as often happens) and the baby is frustrated ; and as for the relationship between the embryo and the male parent, as Samuel Butler said :

D

" A man first quarrels with his father about three-quarters of a year before he is born. It is then he insists on setting up a separate establishment." (14).

Not only are early so-called death-wishes void of any real death-significance, but it is also doubtful whether they lead to the earliest apprehension of the idea. The impressions given by the behaviour of the children observed during this research suggests that the idea arises independently of the earlier impulses towards aggression, and is only linked up with such impulses and flooded with the emotions connected with them at a later stage of development. This point is discussed more fully in Chapters VI and VII.

But if we find that the idea of death does not arise directly from so-called death-wishes, that is not to say that it arises independently of any emotional impulse. It is rather to insist that impulses do not condition intellectual development in such a piecemeal way. The intellect advances like a mighty tide, impelled by the whole surge of the life-impulse ; interests arise, percepts are integrated, ideas are understood, as the tide advances, because it has reached the point when it is ready to engulf them. Particular impulses make a difference, but only so much as the difference between the ebb and flow of the margin waves ; very little in relation to the tide. Receiving and shaping this great natural advance stands the innate constitution of the individual, the bed-rock that is inborn personality.

If therefore we find (as we do find later) that the idea of death develops in the individual as his intellect advances, rather than as his mere years increase or his personal experience teaches ; if we find that the concept of death includes much which a mere becoming-conscious of a death-wish would never suggest—we are not thereby denying a creative relationship between the erotic impulse and the concept of death. We are tracing, rather, the relationships of the deepest currents of emotion and intellect.

It is necessary to stress this because it may be suggested that the concept of death originates in, or is in some way closely related by origin to, either the " death-wish " or the " death-instinct." But when we are considering the origins of intellectual processes, we may set the death-instinct on one side. As Freud described it, it surely cannot be a source of conceptual thought. It is the principle leading away from thought, and from every form of active organization of life. Every thought activity depends on active biological organization. The idea of death, like every other product of thinking, represents an organized activity, a positive biological progress ; it is a functioning and a furtherance of life. An instinctual urge to disintegrate can have no part in producing such a manifestation.

This has led us far from the actual fantasies of actual children. When we come to the study of the thing itself we are faced with the question : Do children spontaneously bring death into their fantasies ? Do they think about it much, of their own will, or is it usually forced upon their notice ? Are most old fairy-stories unsuitable for children, because they are too lurid and too gruesome ?

Two parents who were both psychologists (Drs. D. and R. Katz) (35.i) wrote on this subject :

" We tried in every way to keep from our children the idea of the death of people, and we believe that a similar reticence (is) common to most parents. . . . It is true that in fairy-tales there is a great deal—indeed too much—about striking dead, burning to death, hanging and other methods of causing the transition from life to death, but the child does not comprehend what really lies behind it. For the child, death in fairy-tales probably means nothing more than ' not playing any longer,' the withdrawal of the person concerned. Our children also spoke quite often about murder and shooting in the shallow sense just mentioned."

This passage has value as an illustration of adult attitudes, and it will be referred to again in that connection later (in Chapter V). But only the last sentence gives evidence of the children's actual behaviour. Whatever death may have meant to these children it certainly was not absent from their thoughts.

The clearest witness to the same fact was given in the Geneva report on the Story-Completion Test, already mentioned. Mdlle. Thomas there wrote :

" Nous avons été frappé en dépouillant nos résultats, de trouver traité très fréquemment, soit dans les rêves, soit dans les fantaisies, soit directement, un sujet absolument étranger à nos histoires ; *la mort* (66% des cas) " (71.ii).

Would this result be repeated with other children ? Would it be repeated if the test was not used purposely to unravel children's emotional tangles, but simply to record their immediate fantasy-reactions ?

In substance the result was repeated. In our story-openings, as in Mdlle. Thomas's, there was of course no reference whatever to death. We reduced her material a little, and followed up responses probably much less. Even so, out of 98 children tested, 45 referred to death, funerals, killing or ghosts, in their completions of the stories, and a further five did so spontaneously during the test interview. Ten children who made no explicit reference to it may have been speaking of death when they used phrases by which it is often popularly referred to, such as " She *lost* one of her children," or when they spoke of accidents, as " He got run over."

Thus the most rigid scoring gave 46 per cent for children who made such references in fantasy, 51 per cent when we include those who made spontaneous references of some kind, and 60 per cent was the number when ambiguous cases were included.

Obviously it is impossible that children should think

about death *less* than they speak about it. And since these story-openings present the children with situations which they can and do immediately envisage in terms of their own daily life, the results certainly suggest that the thought of death comes readily to their minds.

But the insight given into their thoughts on this subject by their responses cannot be adequately represented by numbers or percentages. To illustrate something of its quality, and also the method of scoring, some of the responses to story 5 which brought in death either explicitly or doubtfully, are given below. Those reckoned in the 46 per cent are marked (Yes).

SOME COMPLETIONS OF STORY 5[1] FROM ORDINARY-SCHOOL
CHILDREN

Name	*Age*	*Response*
John D.	11 : 7	Because she hadn't enjoyed herself—perhaps they'd lost one of their children, miss.
Edna K.	11 : 1	Because the little girl was very ill and the mother was sad because of another reason. The father got in a smash and he was dead so she had only her little girl and now this poor little girl nearly died. The lady ran for a doctor and a nurse and a lot more doctors. They cured the little girl but she was never properly better—she died at convalescent, and the lady she went silly, and that was why she was so unhappy. (Yes.)
Iris G.	10 : 1	Because one of their children had got drifted out to sea and she couldn't get her back.

[1] Story-opening 5 : One Sunday the boy (or, they all) went out for the day with his (their) father and mother. When they came home in the evening the mother was very sad. Why?

Derrick F.	9 : 11	Because somebody might've died in the family. (Yes.)
George P.	9 : 5	She lost her little boy. He fell in the water and drowned. (Yes.)
Betty M.	9 : 0	One of her little girls had got lost.
Anthony C.	8 : 10	Because she'd lost her boy.
Patricia K.	8 : 4	Because she'd lost one of her children. (How?) The child was paddling in the water, and a great big fish came up and ate her. (Yes.)
Peter T.	8 : 4	P'r'aps one of 'er ba . . . p'r'aps one of 'er little children was gone—they might've gone down a ditch in a pond or a river. (Yes.)
Fred L.	7 : 7	'Cos 'er girl was dead—or 'er boy. (Yes.)
Bill H.	7 : 0	Because the children had got run over, or fell over and hurt their knee.
Josie I.	7 : 0	Because the father—because somebody might have died down there, the father or anybody. (Yes.)
Ted E.	4 : 8	Because her little boy died. (Yes.)

Now the question arises, whether one or more of the story-openings gives such a strong suggestion of the idea of death as to make its completion with some reference to death a matter of conventional closure. For although, if this were so, the number of such references would still give some evidence that the idea comes readily to children's minds and may often be expressed without resistance, yet it would obviously be less significant than if it were found as the response to a variety of different stimuli, and if the responses were of a highly individual character.

Undoubtedly the latter is the case. It can be shown that this is so by comparing the death references with the even more numerous references to punishment, and by examining also their diversity in type.

The idea of punishment occurs in the responses of 65 children (as against 60 at most with the death references). Fifty-five of these children referred to punishment in their completion of story 2. In fact, that story provides something in the nature of a conventional stimulus for the idea of punishment ; six out of every ten children, on an average, completed it with a punishment *motif*. None of the stories seem to provide a conventional stimulus for the idea of death ; story 5 was the nearest, but even when ambiguous references are included, not more than three in ten children, on an average, completed it with a death idea.

Stories 5, 7*b* and 8*b* together account for the majority of the references to death, but such references were liable to appear in any response between 5 and 10 inclusive. One child even brought in a thought of death when she was planning how to spend a fortune (see Josie I., below), but in this she was singular. The first response given below was also unique of its kind. But actually, including these, we find that some reference to death might occur in the completion of any story-opening after the first three. This suggests that familiarity with the test situation and a general sense of mental ease may have been factors as important as any particular suggestion contained in the story-openings themselves.

EXAMPLES OF CHILDREN'S REFERENCES TO DEATH IN RESPONSE
TO DIFFERENT STORY-OPENINGS

Name and Age	" *Normal* " or *Clinic*		*Story Number and Response*
Pamela Q. 10 : 11	C.	4.	They wanted to get rid of their children.
,, ,,	,,	,, 5.	Because she had lost something . . . or perhaps somebody died ?

George K. 9 : 3 N. 6. (Long silence, then speech rather hurried and indistinct) . . . don't mind saying . . . a boy just say . . . that his mother was dead.

Margaret C. 4 : 8 N. 7a. " Snow White. I heard her on the wireless but I haven't seen her (*i.e.*, at ' the pictures '). I've seen her dead, there, in a story book, and going to live with the Prince. I said a picture of her dying, and it's a picture of her dead ! They were lovely pictures ! "

Lily O. · 10 : 5 N. 7a. About someone would come in her room and kill her.

" " " " 7b. Like someone in her family might have died or gone away in hospital while she was in bed.

Ralph O. 10 : 3. N. 8a. He dreamed that somebody had been took off in a lonely lane and when they found him he went to be hanged. (Said in a low, hurried voice.)

Albert I. 10 : 1 C. 8b. A burglar had got in his window and took all the things away and smashed up the home and killed his mother and father.

" " " " 9. His mother and father to come back to life again ; and to have his home back ; and all the furniture and stuff back.

Bert D.	9 : 8	N.	10.	(When grown up, wants to be) " An air pilot. My uncle used to be a pilot but 'e got killed—in a crash—'e was only young. . . . Rough landing . . . petrol clock tank empty . . . before he could jump to safety, the plane crashed. It was only by luck 'e got this job of flying," . . . etc.
Desmond I.	9 : 6	N.	10.	" Said he wanted to stop a boy, so that (*i.e.*, because) as he grows older there is less life in him."
Josie I.	7 : 0	N.	11.	Save it, and buy somefink nice—a present for 'er mother—or a bunch of flowers to put on 'er father's grave.[1]

It may be suggested that the surprising frequency of death references is due to another possible source of error. Some of the responses were made by " ordinary school " children (such as those marked " N " in the above examples) and some by children seen in clinics. When we reckoned up the total number of death references, these two groups were not distinguished. Did this lead to an over-estimate of the readiness of children to think about death, through an over-loading of the total with clinical cases—" problem children " —who might be more subject to anxieties on this subject ? There is no reason to suppose so, for when the clinical children are considered separately it is found that the proportion who refer to death in their responses is actually lower than the total score ; namely, 12 cases in 25, or 48 per cent, as against 51 per cent in the total number of cases.

Another criticism on quite different lines may be made.

[1] Josie's father is not dead. See also her response, p. 38.

It may be suggested that the frequency of the idea of death in these children's responses is simply due to the fact that the test leads to the expression of emotional complexes, as it was specifically designed to do.

In one sense this is true. We have purposely provided the child with a frame in which he can express emotional attitudes which he does not frequently get an opportunity to express in ordinary school or home converse. But if it is implied by this that the idea of death, being one of a very limited number of concepts present in the deeper strata of mind, is necessarily brought to the surface because we are dredging, as it were, when we give this test, then there is a certain misapprehension. The psychologist does not in a single interview break through all those veils of repression which the psychotherapist takes months or years to pierce. The responses provide rich material surprisingly quickly, but mental processes of which the child is unconscious do not immediately at this stimulus leap into the light of day fully clothed, in words all made to fit, each word-concept suited to its appropriate unconscious concept. Word-symbols for death do not lead back to one correlative concept in the unconscious mind. They lead back to a meaning-complex into which many, perhaps all, unconscious concepts are woven. These unconscious concepts are in all very few, and it may be that all meanings are ultimately but different patternings woven from them. Even if there be an unconscious concept of " dead " (which is doubtful), these children, when they use the word, may not be representing that concept ; they might be interpreted as representing with the words " dead," " killed," etc., unconscious ideas of castration, impotence, birth—in fact, almost any other of the limited unconscious group which their minds have woven into the individual meaning-complex for death. And on the other hand, their " death-wishes " may not be expressed in terms of these words at all.

It is not, therefore, because the range of concepts in the

unconscious mind is limited, and death is one of them, that we have so many references to death when we tap children's emotional complexes. It is rather because, when fantasy-thought is stirred, almost any of these unconscious concepts may give rise to a thought of death.

Death, whatever it may mean to children, comes readily into their fantasy thought. So much we may conclude from the evidence of the Story-Completion Tests in Geneva and in London. But when we turn to consider what it does mean to them, we seem at first to reach a *reductio ad absurdum*, a rootlessness of the idea, since it may represent some quite different idea from itself, which again may not be the same in different people, or in the same people at different times. And our material gives very inadequate clues as to what, even in any single case, these deeper ideas may be.

The absurdity, however, is more apparent than real. It arises from a false or partial conception of *meaning*, due to over-emphasis on components that have special importance for the psychotherapist. In every individual the pattern of all meanings is probably laid down in the ways the earliest concepts are interwoven, by the play of conflicting or co-operating impulses. When impulses are obstructed at an early stage of development, they may give rise to concepts which do not play their proper part in the forming or the functioning of the meaning-complexes. These concepts, outlawed, appear to maintain an existence independent of the larger mental developments in which they are forbidden to participate, and from their brigand haunts they exercise a morbid influence on thought and behaviour. It follows that they come to be considered by the therapist as the meaning, *par excellence*, of such thoughts and such behaviour. And in consequence the concepts which arise from early impulses, even when they play their normal part in mental development, come to be considered as ultimate meanings of later processes. But actually, behind every conscious idea there is operative a meaning not expressible in the terms or symbols of one stage only of mental development, but built up and integrated from the experience of every stage and functioning as a whole, in the way (to return to our earlier analogy) in which a violin may function, not always with every string sounding at once, yet never as though its parts were unconnected.

So even when we do not know what are the more primitive relevant concepts and patterns of thought in the individual's experience, we may still validly use as material everything relevant that comes to hand from his later behaviour in seeking to discover the meaning of death for him. And indeed, when we have not the chance of constant, intimate contact with the subject—which is to say, whenever we wish to study a considerable number of subjects simultaneously—we shall probably be on sounder ground if we make the fullest possible use of what is immediately and directly given, than if we seek to reduce it to matter more primitive and remote, since this can only be properly done in the light of extensive and intimate knowledge of each individual mentality.

The question of the early patterning of primitive concepts in forming the idea of death will therefore be deferred to the later chapters (mainly VII and VIII) where an account is given of the behaviour of children in their own homes. The reactions of the hundred-odd school children are considered more in cross-section.

Viewing them in this way, one notices, first that the stimulus which arouses the death-idea provides evidence as to that idea's meaning, as significant as the content of the response itself, since the stimuli—the story-openings—made no direct reference to the idea. As already noted, although the idea of death might appear in any response after the third, there was appreciable clustering around certain openings (stories 5, 7b, 8b). The stimuli presented in these story-openings are evidently suggestions of sorrow and of fear. They are not general suggestions of these emotions, but particularized to certain situations : the sorrow suggested is first, that of a mother, then that of a child lying in bed at bed-time ; the fear is that of a child waking in the night.

The child who responds to these story-stimuli with an idea of death, almost always follows a certain typical pattern in his response. The mother's sorrow is because she has *lost* her child or children. The child's sorrow is because he has *lost* a parent, or both parents. It is a sorrow about death conceived as separation or loneliness. The fear, on the other hand, is not simply of death ; it is of an aggressive outsider (a " burglar ") breaking into the home and killing the child, and perhaps his parents, too. It is a fear of death conceived as the ultimate effect of aggression, violation and robbery.

Thus against the background in which it most commonly appears spontaneously in childish fantasy, death is seen as a typical sorrow-bringing thing and a typical fear-bringing thing.

These two themes, of death as sorrowful separation and of death as the ultimate result of aggression, stand out as the main typical connotations of the idea by whatever method we have studied it. We trace them not so much through the direct word-responses of the children, as by the context in which they produce a response that has reference to death. We shall trace them again in the more detailed studies of individual reactions, and shall then suggest certain links that may exist between the two themes, in the child's early mental development. But at the stage at which we study the idea of death, the duality is a very clear one.

The content of the children's responses gives elaborations and variations on each theme. When the idea of death appears in the context of the mother's sorrow, there is very frequently the suggestion that the child was drowned. This was probably partly a result of the special circumstances of the main group of children, to whom an excursion of the whole family suggested a trip to the seaside. But psycho-analysis suggests that to the unconscious mind, death by drowning implies an identification of life after death with pre-natal life in the womb. The same applies to death by being swallowed up. It appears probable that in some at least of these children's fantasies, these unconscious identifications played a considerable part. For example, Patricia K., aged eight, said the mother was sad because " the child was paddling in the water, and a great big fish came up and ate her." Then, in a later response, Patricia's mother " heard someone crying in the bedroom, and it was a lovely new baby for her, and the same name as the other little girl." Here we see clearly the association of death with pre-natal life, and the logical conclusion of that identification in the rebirth of the same person. Occasionally the association of death with drowning, and the suggestions or womb-symbolism, occur in other contexts ; Freddie, for instance, feared that the burglar who killed him would put his body in a sack and throw it in the river.

The frightening burglar and the body in the sack are familiar fantasies to the psychologist who treats children at clinics. A variation of fantasy involving the idea of death which was also common but more unexpected was the *bird's-nesting* theme. If this had appeared mainly in the responses of the country boys one would not have been surprised ; but some of the most significant fantasies were given by town boys, and some by town girls. In several children's responses, the impression was given that the Freudian Œdipus-complex was being expressed in fantasy form in these terms. The bird in the nest with the eggs symbolizes clearly the human mother and her young ones, or her fertility ; and birds are peculiar among animals in the devotion of the male parent to the female and the young. For children, the ordinary animal family cannot symbolize their whole conflict, because the main source of that conflict —the presence of the male parent, rivalling the child in the mother's attention—is absent among most mammals. This may be why birds find such an important place in children's fantasy ; a place often larger than the child's actual activity in bird's-nesting appears to justify, and a place which may partly account for the common childish passion for bird's-nesting (particularly among boys) and many of its associated phenomena.

An example of the development of the idea of death in association with this bird's-nesting symbolism was found in the case of George D., a very intelligent boy (I.Q. 129) of nine years, seen at a clinic ; a boy of sound general physique and slow, thoughtful manner, suffering from the physical and psychological consequences of an early mastoid operation which had left him completely deaf in one ear, and had separated him from his home for a considerable period at five years of age.

George D. : Story-completions (For test see p. 16).

6. (The other boy told him a secret, namely :) He had been cruel to a bird and taken its nest away and by accident dropped the eggs and broken them. But the boy liked animals, and told his mother, who told the boy's mother.

7a. (In bed at night he thought :) About the trouble he had got into for breaking the bird's nest—his mother told him that to the birds he was like a giant.

7b. He had dreamed that a giant had taken him away, and he knew it was God's punishment for breaking the eggs, and he never did such a cruel thing again.

8b. For the dream had frightened him so much he cried out for his mother, and then he said he was only dreaming and it was about giants.

9. (For his three wishes :) He wished that animals would like him, and that he would never break an egg again, and that he would always be kind to dogs—to weak creatures.

10. (He wished :) To stay a child always . . . to play with birds and dogs—and friends as well.

11. (With £100,000 :) He bought lots of kinds of animals—had a bird-haven, and a beast-haven, and people

came to buy eggs from the creature-haven, and one of his hens laid a golden egg . . . pure gold, and he could spend it.

Q. : What did he spend it on ?

George : On more hens.

The unconscious mind is very fond of puns, and I think George's " bird-haven and beast-haven," his " creature-haven," is really Heaven. There, all the animals belong to him, and one of the hens produces a specially precious egg, which is his own valuable property, yet cannot be put to more happy use than to produce more of its own kind, more hens, for George.

In George's fantasies we find a variation on the childish attitude to the death-idea, which has not yet been touched upon. It is implied by him, as by other children in their burglar-fantasies, that death is the effect of aggression. But with George the emotional knot is uncovered also at an earlier twist : it is his own aggressiveness that brings about the accident. It is his own cruelty which arouses in him nightmareish fears of punishment ; punishment on talion principles, by God, by a giant, who takes *him* away from *his* home-nest, just as he, acting giant-like, took the eggs away.

Further analysis might show more fully what the eggs represent to the child—the male (his own or his father's) potential sexual activity, or the female's ; or babies as rivals to himself. The responses in themselves show how being " taken away " by God is a retaliation-punishment (that is to say, is equated with) taking away and destroying a nest and eggs (fertility). Killing and dying have thus become part of a complex which is evidently Œdipal in its nature.

The connection of the complex with the mother is also made clear by George himself. It is his mother who shows him his identification with the giant and warns him of danger ; it is his mother to whom he turns for protection against the giant, as the baby bird would turn to the hen.

And we see how naïvely, in George's fantasies, he derives his kindliness to his fellows from his fear of punishment. Finally, he does take the " creatures " away, but reconciles himself to this realization of his desires (and his retaliation fears) by treating the animals with kindness, making the place a " haven." The spectre of guilt is laid ; his hens now belong to him, and lay eggs which are his to spend, without stealing. Beyond hens and property in eggs there is nothing to desire, but more hens.

DEATH AND TALION

In George's fantasies the idea of death is clearly implicit, but what it means to the child can only be appreciated when his responses are considered as a whole. The significance is to be found not so much in any particular identification of one idea with another, nor even in a particular content of thought, but rather in a manner of thinking. An oscillation of circumstance leads George to be " taken away," and later leads the birds who were at first his victims into their " haven."

Again and again in the children's responses we find together the idea of death as result of aggression, and this mental oscillation. The oscillation in their fantasies is often expressed in typical terms of talion, when all happens tit-for-tat ; but at times the oscillation seems more fundamental than the talion theme, and more fundamental than the idea of guilt which is also the common accompaniment of the idea of death-as-aggression.

The impression is given that the idea of retaliation itself, primitive as it is, develops from a manner of thought still more general and primitive. This manner of thought is an oscillation of attention, by which a whole fantasy or thought-complex is alternately seen in primary and then in reversed aspect, and then again in primary. Thus, a mother loses her child by death, and then the mother herself dies ; and

E

then the child (or a substitute) is alive again ; and then the mother comes back, too.

As a mental process, this oscillation of attention in fantasy shows parallels with that oscillation[1] of attention in perception which has been investigated in psychological laboratories. In the laboratory we find that if we fix our eyes on a pattern of dots or a figure in ambiguous perspective, after a time the pattern changes before our eyes, independently of our volition, and after going through one or more such changes, returns to the original phase ; and this process will continue so long as we maintain our attention on the same object. In the oscillations of fantasy, however, the phenomenon is complicated by the fact that each phase is to some extent affected by the experiences that precede it. Thus, if a mother loses her child by death (primary phase), there is a suggestion of remorse associated with her own death (secondary phase) ; the birth of another child or of some substitute involves reparation and forgiveness, so that we revert to the primary phase but with richer connotations ; and the mother, or her motherhood, can now return to make everything just and right (secondary phase).

It is as though the oscillations of fantasy gather cumulative force. In both fantasy and sensory perception, however, the completion of the second phase appears to bring the adjustment of a balance which the first phase has upset. With sensory perception, this readjustment may be conceived in physiological terms. In fantasy it is commonly expressed in terms of ethics. " Tit-for-tat," children cry ; or if one boy hits another, and the first hits back, they say, " It serves you *right.*" " An eye for an eye, a tooth for a tooth," is typical primitive justice ; " give and take " is a precept of social

[1] To distinguish it from oscillation in work-output, oscillation of attention is now more properly designated " fluctuation." I am indebted to Mr. S. de Alvis for this information, but I think it unfortunate that the terms are not used in the reverse way.

ethics that strikes home to the simplest mind. Young children
can be persuaded reluctantly to cease a fruitless struggle for
conflicting joys by the suggestion to "take it in turns"; they
are able to recognize an elementary justice in this.

Where fantasy or actual behaviour thus oscillate over a
basic pattern, the figures which take each other's place
become mentally identified. (In the parallel case with
sensory perception the figures *are* identical, and it is fantasy
alone that makes distinctions between them.) This generalization is, of course, an over-simplification of the situation,
perhaps a reversal of the time-order of the mental processes
involved. It may be that an impulse towards identification
—a desire to be a substitute—causes the original pattern to
form in the mind, and starts the movement of oscillation.
Thus, the child desires to take the father's place, and have
the mother for his wife. In fantasy he identifies himself with
the father ; their positions then begin to oscillate. But with
each oscillation, new emotional complications are carried
forward from the last phase. So guilt arises subsequently to
the identification of the child with his father and a complete
oscillation of the pattern ; the guilt is compounded of his
desire for his mother seen from his point of view as child and
from his point of view as father.

It is not intended to suggest that the sense of guilt must
necessarily derive from this particular fantasy-pattern. The
child may at a very early stage experience oscillation of the
mother-child-feeding situation in fantasy, and exchange
positions with his *mother*. Infants barely weaned, long before
they can walk or talk, may be seen spontaneously to offer
their biscuit to their mother to eat. Hence a child refusing
his food may, on this basis, feel guilt.

The whole process has great significance in connection
with the development of the idea of death. It has a double
significance, for first it has that which is common to the
development of all forms of meaning. The emotional
impulses behind any conception lead, in each case, through

identifications based on desire, to oscillations of attention and aspect, and a continually widening synthesis. But these identifications and oscillations are particularly significant for the idea of death, because the idea has an utterly different connotation when it is attached to the self, from that which it has when attached to other people. This point, however, cannot be properly developed here, for its illustration depends on the record of reactions of the children more intimately known.

The oscillatory process may be illustrated from the children's story-completion fantasies, first through an example which does not involve death, but is strong in the idea of retaliation, and then by one which does involve death but leaves the retaliation idea implicit. Freddie G. (8 : 8), in the person of the story boy, was told by one of his friends the secret that " he knocked some boy out, and people didn't know who'd done it. But (Freddie) went and let it out on him." Then (Freddie) thought " about the boy who told him about knocking out the boy." And he felt sad because " he hurt himself." Then (Freddie) dreamed " about the boy knocking *him* out " ; and he was frightened because " the boy was just about to knock him out, and he woke up with the fright." So, given a wish, he asked for a pair of boxing-gloves. Edna L., a miserable, under-nourished-looking girl of seven, gave these responses :

(The mother was sad :) 'Cos the father died.
(In bed at night the little girl thought :) Somebody was coming in 'er 'ouse.
7b. (The little girl was sorry :) 'Cos 'er father died.
Q. : What happened then ?
Edna : She died 'erself.
8a. (She dreamed :) That somebody walked in 'er 'ouse and made 'er frightened.
9. (She wished, from the fairy :) That 'er father would come alive again.

Q. : And then? (Edna only having given one instead of three wishes).

Edna : A little pony.

The law of talion is represented at many different levels of social behaviour, from the impulsive returning of blow for blow that may occur among animals at play, to the vicarious sacrifice symbolized by the Eucharist. Between retaliation and sadism or sheer violence (whether rationally or irrationally directed) there is an absolute and clear distinction : retaliation seeks to right a balance ; it presupposes a supporting framework which includes both parties and it is itself a function of the whole, concerned with the maintenance of the whole in equilibrium. The liberty, equality and fraternity of man are all concerned in retaliation. Retaliation can be no function of the subservient, and only those equal in spirit and impulse can gain in grace by voluntarily refraining from it.

Retaliation is, then, a fundamentally ethical procedure. But the fact that it takes place within a social framework implies much more. For this social framework is built up on identification of the component parts. The process of oscillation which retaliation represents in the legal-ethical field involves reversability of the functions of its members, as automatically as the figure in ambiguous perspective presents first one aspect of itself and then another. This involves for each participator a fundamental duality of parts, and mental conflict. Each feels himself at once avenger and victim. For in each mind the succeeding phases leave their cumulative deposits of emotion, and no attitude completely succeeds the last, or reverts to a form identical with an earlier one.

Thus it is not merely a brilliant ingeniousness on the part of the victim which suggests his offering reparation before he has it forced upon him by the avenger. He does not only represent himself, nor himself in the circumstances of this occasion alone. He represents both wrongdoer and wronged within himself, with an alternation similar to that which maintains primitive society. Since these alternations in fantasy-processes are not simple and discrete, but cumulative, retaliation in practice rarely results in an endless ding-dong of revenge, but gives place to a system of reparation which has its foundation not in forcible imposition, but in the deeper social sense, and hence the acquiescence, of the wrong-doer and the wronged.

In the children's responses to the Story-Completion Test the talion process can be seen at work at different levels of development. Freddie G.'s responses, already quoted, show a fairly primitive type of retaliatory attitude, with considerable uncertainty and complexity of identification. In Edna's responses one observes the spirit of reparation rather than retaliation. After she has imagined her father dead she imagines herself dead—this is reparation, not retaliation, for it is not that her father kills her, or that his ghost frightens her. Then she wishes him alive again, in fantasy ; and then, " a little pony." This little pony I believe to be Edna herself reborn ; the clearer cases of such transformation, in support of this theory, must be deferred till later.

George's responses in their sequence illustrate the ethical development of talion law. His murderous behaviour is avenged on him in identical form ; he, the new victim, recognizes this as " God's punishment," and hence just. He seeks the forgiveness of his own victims, and finally attempts to make a complete reparation to them by securing their perpetual happiness through his own benevolence.

Thus we see that as fantasy oscillates, and accumulates from each phase emotional attitudes and identifications which are carried over to the next, new syntheses arise, and more comprehensive contrasts appear. Simple antagonisms at first work themselves out in blow for blow, until the complications of identification make victory or loss for either into victory or loss for both ; and then these alternating phases are seen as a single phase of conflict and killing, and another phase appears, to contrast with the first one as a whole. Mutual-hate-and-murder gives place to mutual-love-and-resurrection.

Edna's father is not dead. If he were, would it make a difference to her fantasies? How does the child think about death, in his fantasies, if one of his family has actually died recently?

Then we do in some cases notice a difference. There may then be no mention of death at all, but the idea of guilt may assume obsessional proportions in the content of the child's thought. He may express a fear of imprisonment, and see every misfortune of himself or anyone else as a just punishment, from which he assumes that they have been guilty of some crime, although he may have no idea what the crime could be.

The clearest example of this process at work was given by Bernard N., a curly-haired, healthy-looking little boy of 8 : 2. So strong and all-pervasive were Bernard's reactions to his father's death that they appeared in his responses from beginning to end of the test-situation, not only in the Story-Completion Test. To begin with, he was not prepared to give his surname, now that his father was dead. The experimenter thought at first that perhaps he was an illegitimate child, and then that perhaps his mother had re-married, but this was not so. Perhaps his hesitation arose from the fact that his name came from his father, and now that he had no father he was doubtful whether he still had the name. But more probably the explanation is given in his own response to problem IX.2b, next page.

Bernard was very ready to talk about the sad event as it actually happened in his experience, but no mention of death appears in his fantasies. They are full of aggressive ideas, however, while his consciously-directed thinking is full of the fear of imprisonment and a sense of guilt, which he imports into every situation presented. He is afraid of growing bigger. His dearest wish is for a magic wand, to " change an animal into a man, a real man." We may compare Edna's little pony ; Bernard's animal-man is, I think, the father re-created.

Bernard's actual responses are given below. The interview occurred on 3rd March, 1938, when the children of London had no thought of war as touching their own homes or families : it will be remembered that this was a few days before the German Government annexed Austria, six months before they annexed Czecho-Slovakia, eighteen months before they invaded Poland and Great Britain declared war. To London children at that time actual hostilities were very remote.

Bernard N., 8 : 2

    E. : What's your name ?
    B. : Bernard.
    E. : And your other name ?
    B. : Don't know.
    E. : What's your Mummie's name ?
    B. : Mrs. (N.).
    E. : And your Dad ?
    B. : 'Aven't got a dad.
    E. enquired about the number in the family. B. said there were eight of them, and then went on :
    B. : There would have been nine if my Dad was alive. . . . 'E died up Kennington Park. 'E was so glad 'e 'ad the baker's job, and 'e was ill of a night, and 'e fell down and a policeman (came and told the mother he had died). My mum was crying. . . .

INTELLIGENCE TEST RESPONSES

    IX.2*b*. (" Absurdity " problem : " A man called one day at the post office and asked if there was a letter waiting for him. ' What is your name ? ' asked the postmaster. ' Why,' said the man, ' you will find my name on the envelope.' ")

B. : He didn't tell him his name . . . he wouldn't tell him his name, because he didn't want to be put away and put in the police station.

VII.4a. (Comprehension problem : " What's the thing for you to do when you have broken something which belongs to someone else ? ")

B. : Get put away in a home . . . where all the other naughty boys go.

IX.2d. (Absurdity problem : " In an old graveyard they have discovered a small skull which they believe to be that of (Nelson) when he was about ten years old.")

B. : 'Cos 'e was fighting when 'e was ten years old. Because 'e shouldn't go to fight. Because 'e shouldn't 'ave joined the army.

Definition of obedience : " When you don't disobey God."
Definition of dead : " When your father's dead."

STORY-COMPLETION RESPONSES

7a. (He thought) that there was going to be a war. That he may get put in prison.

7b. (He was sad) 'cos somebody may 'ave 'it 'im or pinched 'im.

8b. (He was frightened) 'cos there may have been somebody in the 'ouse.

9. (He wished for) a magic wand. To change all the things into different things. Changed an animal into a man, a real man.

10. (He wished) to stay little. Because 'e didn't like it when 'e was grown up. He tried to make himself smaller.

No direct mention of death appeared in Bernard's fantasies, though his conversation showed how much the idea was on his mind. Similar reticences have been observed by other students of childhood. Dr. Ruth Griffiths (23.i) tells of one of the children she studied, who was full of aggressive ideas and death-wishes against her sister. The father had already died, and also a friend called Dorothy. When the sister (whose name was also Dorothy) became ill, and the child's death-wish against her sister seemed to be approaching realization, she ceased to express it. Richard Hughes, in his brilliant study, *A High Wind in Jamaica*, describes how, when one of the children (they were all far from home, among strangers) died a sudden, violent death, the others simply ceased to refer to him, and behaved as though he had never been. This is very much the way the children behave in the Story-Completion Test ; that is to say, when they are participating in fantasy-thought, they avoid all reference to death if someone closely connected with them has recently died.

But this is not the way they behave with adults in ordinary intercourse. They are ready to talk about the matter to a friendly adult ; they volunteer it (the experimenter was entirely ignorant of Bernard's family affairs, until he told her) ; they may even show themselves anxious to talk things over in this more " rational " way.

Why is this ?

To understand the conflict in the child's mind at such a time, we must take account of a factor which we have as yet overlooked : his conception of causality. It would be an over-simplification to say that the child believes in his own *omnipotence*, in the sense that he believes that his wishes take effect automatically. Undoubtedly his mental scheme includes a variety of forms of causation, with little co-ordination between them. But it is a characteristic feature of the thought of the child, that his own wishes have magical power to influence events. From his babyhood he preserves an impression of himself as the activating centre of his world, whose wishes are known, carried out or thwarted, even when he does not or cannot express them. So it happened with him in babyhood, apparently ; so, he more than half believes, it continues to happen.

Consequently, in the child's fantasy, he takes responsibility for his wishes. Unconscious logic works ruthlessly in both directions. If things don't happen, then he didn't wish them. If things do happen, then it was because he wished them. If his father or little sister have died, that is because he wished it. He must have wished it. So he is responsible for it.

An actual death among those near him emotionally thus proves to the child the comparative weakness of his own love-impulses (or the general malevolence of fate) ; and through the child's identification of himself with the dead person it proves the same hatred in him. It proves, also, the dead one's power to harm and kill. The child may begin to suffer from nameless anxiety, or from fear of ghosts. If he is at a stage of simple retaliation-fantasy he will fear punishment, such as imprisonment for murder ; if, on the other hand, he has come to the stage of reparation in fantasy, he may become over-obedient and conscientious.

From this painful situation the child may make what psycho-analysts have called a flight into reality. That is, he represses (normally only for a time) all fantasy about death, and limits his thought about it to what can be expressed in terms of the socially-determined, generally accepted, adult attitude. This adult attitude involves a complete rejection of the whole idea of the child's personal responsibility for the death in question. The notion of magical power and personal responsibility fits in with the limited world-pattern of a baby whose fantasy-population includes but two or three protagonists, and whose ethics are simple talion. But in the adult world-pattern, the population is expanded to include mankind, and the ethics implied are those of mutual fellowship and responsibility.

Such a pattern (that is to say, such a conception of reality) is the resultant of a long process of cumulative syntheses in thought which the child cannot immediately experience directly as his own. But by suggestion and tradition he can

receive some of their virtue, as indeed he does all through
his life. In contact with an adult he receives the unspoken
assurance that he is not to blame for the death. He is helped
to feel comparatively powerless and unimportant, and so to
shed his belief in his magical powers. It is obvious to the
child that the adult does not completely understand him,
nor automatically know what is going on in his mind. So
he gets assurance that the powers of death may not have
understood or obeyed. Maybe they mistook his orders.
Maybe he never did wish that person to die.

So gradually, helped by the adult's perception of his
innocence and his own perception of how the adult does not
always understand him, the child who has made a " flight
into reality " returns to cultivate his own garden of fantasy.
Gradually he scales down the power and the malevolence
with which he has credited himself, and accepts the
remainder into his scheme without undue repression.

Thus we may reconstruct the reactions and recovery of
the child whose balance has been temporarily upset by the
shock of the death of a near relative.

No two such cases are identical. Among children whose
behaviour was sufficiently normal to arouse no general
comment, Bernard (quoted p. 56) was perhaps an extreme
case, in his " flight into reality " and his sense of guilt.
Ralph O., on the other hand, a country boy aged 9 : 10, had
lost his twin brother as a baby, and whereas he did not avoid
references to death in his fantasies (see p. 40), his behaviour
obviously was far from normal. Among his fellow scouts
he would sometimes burst into tears, and have to be led
from the camp fire by a kindly scoutmaster and comforted ;
but this master did not know why Ralph cried. (As in all
such cases there were other complicating factors in Ralph's
family life.) His death fantasies are distinctly grim, and he
shows a fear of punishment, similar to Bernard's, in the form
of imprisonment. He spoke much of the baby twin, considering he could not remember him, and had other siblings

alive. His three wishes were : " That his . . . that he'd have a happy life, and he wouldn't do anything wrong, and he'd be free."

The case of Irene M., on the other hand (age 7 : 8, I.Q. 100), contrasts strongly with those of both Bernard and Ralph. Her father has recently died, but his brother, a schoolboy only a few years older than Irene, had then come to live with her and her mother, Iiene being the only child. In Irene's fantasies both her mother and her father are disposed of. The mother, having " lost one of her children," herself " might have gone away, or died, or something like that." Then the little girl is made Fairy Queen, but after this she wishes that " if her mother got lost, she would come back again," so long as she herself can remain Fairy Queen and also have her brother for King. (Irene often calls the young uncle her brother.) Thus the mother is quite kindly treated ; the father, on the other hand, is held in absolute contempt. " He went and choked hisself, and the children laughed at him." Later on, " one of them had some money and the father didn't, and they started quarrelling because the little old man wanted some money." It is perhaps not surprising that when the little girl is frightened in the night, " she seen her own shadow, and she thought it was someone in the room, or her father coming in the room and his shadow was on the door, and she was frightened of that." But in general Irene does not seem to suffer from any undue sense of guilt or fear, in the way that Bernard and Ralph do. In fantasy she frankly wants " to grow up . . . and have a little baby," and a direct question on the point of her vocational choice produced only a slight modification of this ; she then answered that she wanted to be a nurse, to nurse babies.

Irene is an interesting phenomenon. Little girls who, in our society, are able to substitute a young lover-uncle for a dead father are rare. It may be a circumstance favourable to the reduction of feminine anxiety.

It seems clear, however, from these cases, that the behaviour of children whose relatives have died may appear peculiar, but nevertheless may be related to the same kind of mental processes and the same background in fantasy, as the thoughts of the unbereaved child with regard to the subject of death.

What then, finally, does death mean in the child's fantasies ? It means separation ; it means the infliction of the extreme of aggression ; it involves grief and fear. But also, as though it were one aspect only of an ambiguous design, death in fantasy continually reverses its appearance, so that the murderer becomes the murdered, and the dead the newly-born.

CHAPTER IV

THE ADULT AND THE CHILD

Sometimes in the course of this winter, my Father and I had long cosy talks together over the fire. Our favourite subject was murders. I wonder whether little boys of eight, soon to go upstairs alone at night, often discuss violent crime with a widower papa? The practice, I cannot help thinking, is unusual; it was, however, consecutive with us. We tried other secular subjects, but we were sure to come round at last to " what do you suppose they really did with the body? " . . . I also heard about Burke and Hare, whose story nearly froze me into stone with horror. . . . I suppose that my interest in these discussions—and Heaven knows I was animated enough—amused and distracted my Father, whose idea of a suitable theme for childhood's ear now seems to me surprising.

(Three years later.) It was at this party . . . that it was proposed that "our young friends" should give their elders the treat of repeating any pretty pieces that they knew by heart. Accordingly a little girl repeated *Casabianca*, and another little girl, *We are seven*. I was then asked. . . . Without a moment's hesitation, I stood forth, and in a loud voice I began one of my favourite passages from Blair's *Grave* :

> If death were nothing, and nought after death—
> If when men died at once they ceased to be,
> Returning to the barren Womb of Nothing
> Whence first they sprung, then might the debauchee. . . .

" Thank you, dear, that will do nicely ! " interrupted the lady with the curls.

EDMUND GOSSE, *Father and Son* (22).

On the question whether adults think much about death, we meet with two opposed schools of thought, based on observations made from different points of view, and each corresponding with certain psychological realities. The existence and opposition of these two viewpoints was neatly illustrated by a recent controversy in *The New Statesman*. The organizers of the sociological studies called Mass-observation, provoked by criticism, turned on their critic, a poet, and suggested that poets are out of touch with the man-in-the-street. The poet had written that

> " A crack in the tea-cup opens
> A lane to the land of the dead."

The Mass-observer objected that for most men it did not. The poet held his ground.

Two American psychologists, Schilder and Wechsler, in a study of *The Attitudes of Children towards Death* (58), refer to opposed views corresponding to those of the mass-observers and the poet : superficial observation suggests, they write, that the majority of human beings do not give much thought to death, throughout the greater part of their lives ; certain introspective philosophers, notably Husserl and Heidegger, suggest the very opposite. Heidegger states that death and absolute nothingness are constantly before the inner eye of man, and that life's inner meaning is derived solely from the ever-present knowledge of inevitable death. He believes that it is through the realization of death that we are enabled to perceive time.[1]

But, as Schilder and Wechsler observe, the matter is not to be decided either by superficial observation or by intro-spection, but by systematic enquiry among a number of subjects, observation and record of their reactions, and the investigation of mental processes both conscious and unconscious.

In an enquiry made in America (50) by the questionnaire method among 825 college students of both sexes, ranging in age from 15 to 24 years, 93 per cent reported that they

---

[1] Heidegger, M., *Sein und Zeit*, quoted by Schilder and Wechsler, *op. cit.* In connection with this view of the relation between the perception of time and the recognition of the inevitability of death the present study is able to offer some observations in Chapter VIII.

thought of their own death very rarely. Fifty-one per cent reported that they made it a practice to attend funeral services infrequently ; another 42 per cent said that they attempted to avoid them altogether. Seventy-eight per cent said that they wished for, and 67 per cent that they believed in, a future existence.

Investigation by means of psycho-analytic technique gave rather different results, though they are not strictly comparable because of the very much smaller number who could be studied. " From such observation it appears that persons who are consciously unconcerned with death are very frequently preoccupied with it in their unconscious life," writes Schilder. Dreams are found to be full of death symbolism and aggressive impulses (" death wishes ") against loved persons. In the adult such fears and wishes are commonly repressed, and there is often deep resistance to their avowal. Bromberg and Schilder give an account of ten cases psycho-analysed with particular reference to " death-wishes " and fears (57.a).

From the results of the questionnaire it would seem that the mass-observers may be justified in supposing that the thought of death rarely appears in the consciousness of the average man. The statement is more likely to be correct if it is limited to the thought of the death of the self. On the other hand the evidence from psycho-analysis suggests and to some extent explains how poets, and possibly some philosophers and others of peculiar bent, may have death constantly in mind, consciously as well as unconsciously. Neurotic obsessions may account for some such cases ; in others it may be attributable to a weaker censorship of these ideas and impulses, or of *id* impulses in general.

From mental strata between those tapped by the questionnaire and by *depth-psychology*, some evidence can also be collected ; namely, from the reading-matter in which the man-in-the-street most indulges. In this we may look for some data as to the character of his predominant fantasies,

F

It will be generally agreed[1] that journals enjoying a particularly large circulation in Great Britain devote a high proportion of their space to accounts of incidents connected with death. If the British public avoided such news-items as frequently and as sedulously as the American students apparently avoid funerals, we should be forced to suppose that the editors supply it with ulterior motives, such as *uplift*, which is unlikely, or that they do not know what pays, which conflicts with the data.

The attraction of these stories is not to be sought in any information they give of general changes in human affairs. They have no *news*-value as such ; their true value comes from what is old and unchanging in them. We may surmise that they provide material for fantasy-identifications similar in kind to those given by the story-openings in the Story-Completion Test ; though the adult readers are provided with more highly suggestive matter, and thereby enabled to repress more deeply the identifications they impress upon it.

The popularity of such journalistic accounts of murder, suicide or other forms of sudden death gives some indication of the frequency of adult thoughts of death at fantasy level, and suggests that it may not be less than that of children, as indicated by the Story-Completion Test.

Do children or adults repress more deeply their thoughts of death ? General observation suggests that adults do so. Instances of children's verbal expression of death-wishes will be given in the home records below (Chapters VI to X).

---

[1] The writer cannot provide evidence for this statement, though she believes it to be correct and to represent a fact. A correlation between size of circulation and space devoted to news-matter about death-incidents would go some way to proving it, but it is obvious that accidental factors might complicate the issue. The conclusion, to be generally valid for psychology, would also need to be based on evidence from many communities. In these communities widespread literacy would be a necessary pre-condition, and also the existence of a popular press financed on a basis of competitive profit-making, free from moral restrictions which might affect the issue.

But in considering the question of whether repression is deeper, one has also to consider the comparative availability of different forms of relief for it, and particularly of the degree and the way in which the maturation of sex and its physical exercise interacts with such repression.

That thoughts about death give rise to anxieties which expression of sexual love may relieve is one of the oldest themes of literature, and finds its clearest demonstration in times of war. But whether the same (or the converse) holds true over long periods of lesser tension is not so apparent. It seems probable that there is some permanent and particular influence, in the normal individual, of the one form of anxiety and expression upon the other, but that the tensions (of death-anxiety and sex) whose simultaneous release is obvious when they are so extreme as to find escape only through crisis (of sexual intercourse, suicide, foolhardy daring, etc.) may when less extreme but enduring be relieved through various aspects of sex or of life-dedication. Shakespeare (60.*a*.i) writes that

" Nothing 'gainst Time's scythe can make defence
Save breed, to brave him when he takes thee hence."

By which he suggests that not the exercise of sexual love but the physical result of it—the reproduction of children—forms a defence, indeed the only defence, against death. It is an attitude so common in the East that its comparative neglect among the peoples of Western culture marks one of the deepest differences between the thought of Orient and Occident. Among the Jews, in religious history and psychological practice, West and East meet ; the traditional functions of the son towards the dead father mark the Eastern attitude ; the development of Christianity marks the Western.

In contrast with this is the tradition of chivalry which derived from the genius of the mediæval Provençal troubadours. An exceedingly elaborate code of sexual love was developed, and used as a defence against death-anxiety. A man's sword and martial endeavour were dedicated to his lady, who, in the true tradition of chivalry, should never be his wife. Indeed, much more than martial endeavour was dedicated to the mistress. Beatrice is Dante's focus for the whole passage through life and eternity. Despite the satire of Cervantes, the same spirit remained alive to be expressed in the lines of Lovelace *To Anthea from Prison* :

> " Bid me to live, and I will live
>   Thy Protestant to be."

His theme is, that he is absolutely free to live, and to love, too, even when stone walls divide him from the lady. Her physical presence is not the essential : his freedom to love her in the spirit is all that is necessary to ensure his freedom from anxiety.

Thus chivalry's mode of using sex-impulses as defence against death-anxiety is in absolute contrast to Shakespeare's in the sonnet quoted. Shakespeare's attitude here is consonant with the idealization of affection between man and man. Such affection contains within itself no defence against death-anxiety. It is therefore properly supplemented by attention to sex in its more purely reproductive aspect. Those who idealize love divorced from sex, and relegate love between the sexes to the lower rank deemed appropriate to its more utilitarian aspect, are often pitifully conscious of the utter helplessness of their emotion in the face of death. These things find expression in an elegy made by the Earl of Surrey for his friend and protégé, Clere. Surrey, soberly recalling Clere's life, records that " in the womb of Ormond's race he bred." Woman could scarcely be more crudely dismissed. But he concludes with the exquisite lament :

" Ah, Clere, if love had counted, care or cost,
    Heav'n had not gained, nor earth so timely lost."[1]

The different ways in which culture has developed and
elaborated the sexual impulse so as to relieve anxieties about
death is an immense subject which can be no more than
touched on here. The point for us is that their efficiency for
the individual is dependent upon his sexual maturity. They
are not genuinely available to the child.

When anxiety about death is aroused in the child, therefore, his mode of defence is likely to be either an escape to
the mental atmosphere of the adult, where safety can be
suggested from sources not available to him when he is
restricted to his own resources, or the use of some mechanism[2]
resembling rather that of a maladjusted adult than of one
for whom his own culture completely fulfils its functions.
These mechanisms attempt a reconciliation to the thought
of death through some other means than those which are
offered by sex and what culture has built upon sex.

One such method is reaction-formation. The sufferer
braves death and takes risks with a foolhardiness not always
apparent as such. Another method is to isolate in consciousness the unpleasant idea (not always one of death) ; this
may cause complete loss of memory for a portion of
experience, or possibly be a factor in bringing on epileptic
attacks. There may be displacement of the affect aroused by
the thought on to something different but associated with

[1] Parallels may be found in the work of A. E. Housman. *Cf.* the
poem beginning " If love, in hearts that perish," and the Epithalamium,
with its reference to the wife as " her who hardly loves you more," and
the injunction to

    " Breed the land that reared your prime
    Sons to stay the rot of time " (29.*b*).

[2] By mechanism is here meant a comparatively elaborate pattern of
behaviour. Repression, projection, introjection would thus not be styled
mechanisms, but would be considered as basic to mechanisms, as running
and kicking are basic to football.

it, or on to some aspect of it from which the unpleasant quality is excluded. This mechanism we shall study later, for in the form of hope of Heaven and fear of Hell it has played a large part in traditional religious forms of relief for death-anxiety. One form of defence does not preclude the use also of another. There may be identification of the self with death personified, together with that oscillation between the parts which has been already studied in children's fantasy thought. Many a human being has taken Death's part, buried his own well-developed personality during life, casting away ambition and worldly goods, often losing his identity so far as he can and changing his name, in his effort to anticipate Death's action against him. As a motive to the monastic life this siding with Death has often been very clear. The Emperor Charles V is the classic instance in history. After his mother's death he always chose hangings of black cloth for his own bedroom ; he abdicated from the rule of a great empire, and in his retirement was intensely preoccupied with funerals, finally celebrating his own while yet alive. The life of T. E. Lawrence provides in our own day an illustration of a similar mechanism at work.

Criminals sometimes attempt to steal a march on Death and the law simultaneously in this way. The law defends its prerogative by taking special precautions against the suicide of the man condemned to death. Other intending suicides may be moved by the desire to cheat not human but natural law of its victim.

Death may be considered as exclusively without or within, projected or introjected. Men may feel it a victory over death to take away his initiative, steal a march on him and do the thing themselves, even when nothing threatens them but the processes of decay. The victim sees outside him a process which is largely within, and then escapes the externalized bogey by reassertion of that very power (the power to die) of which the bogey is but a shadow, an abstraction, Mortality. To such minds the darker and nearer shadow of death that hangs over all in times of war, gives greater power to integrate and assert the personality ; gives them, indeed, vitality and courage.

The normal individual seeks to *guard his ego* in a complex variety of ways ; that is, to keep available for human, social purposes a fund of controllable energy which his own more primitive desires and their resultant anxieties would otherwise swallow up. Sometimes his defences overshoot the mark ; his activities destroy or injure what it is their aim to preserve. Zilboorg (74) has drawn a comparison between certain forms of insanity and suicide, and physiological phenomena observed to occur in cases of peritoneal injury. In an attempt to co-operate, as it were, with the healing process, certain bodily functions are spontaneously suspended ; but at times this suspension is itself excessive, and death ensues from this cause rather than from the injury itself. Similarly, insanity and suicide may be the result of an inability to set again in motion mental processes which have been curatively suspended during crises of reaction to mental injury or stress.

It is obvious that the reactions of the maladjusted adult which involve thoughts of death may be of a kind not readily associated by the adult with childhood. It may be because the adult feels the child to be unable to share in the happier forms of defence against death-anxiety, that he is anxious to shield him from the thought. It is commonly suggested that children never should, and rarely do, think about death. If their interest becomes obvious, the adult reaction is one of surprise, or (among those responsible for the child's mental welfare) of apologetic explanation. This is illustrated in the comments of the Katz's on their children's conversations (35.i). Perhaps a further illustration is to be found in Freud's dismissal of the child's idea of death as equivalent to disappearance or going a journey, and the similar treatment of the theme by Stern.

Dr. Susan Isaacs observed adult reactions to children's

thought about death, when she proposed that children should be taught about sex through biology, and particularly through observation of the behaviour of animals in life, and of their bodies by dissection after they were dead. She notes that "it has not been considered desirable (by public opinion) that the child should take any interest in . . . the facts of death."

" So strong is this widely held attitude," she continues, " that it is difficult to get many people even to consider the possible wisdom of the opposite course. They are too disturbed by the mere suggestion to be able to give it any attention. . . . When one assures them . . . that the majority of little children are neither shocked nor frightened (by ' looking inside ' dead bodies) . . . the solid wall of prejudice does not melt away, and one is in the end left with the suspicion that the real attitude is, ' Well, if they're *not* shocked or frightened, they ought to be ! ' " (33.*a*.i).

Such an attitude, not being founded, as Dr. Isaacs notes, on objective observation of children, must derive from the adult's own wishes and fears. The wish that children should not think about death, arises from the adult's own fear of it ; the erroneous belief that the child does not do so derives from repression of the fear, or more complicated defences against it.

The fear of death is older than the manhood of man ; although in this sense it may be a fear of an unknown. Indeed, in a sense it is always a fear of an unknown, which can only be symbolized, not remembered as an experience.[1]

[1] This statement must be qualified, because of the recollected experiences of those who have actually suffered the biological equivalent of death for a time, and then been revived, by artificial respiration after drowning, or otherwise. One medical man who recounted to the writer his personal experience of this kind (he was functionally lifeless for a considerable time after being severely wounded during the war) stated that he had lost all fear of death as a result of it. His account curiously resembled that of Aeneas when he visited the Elysian fields (*Aeneid*, VI, 637 ff.), except that Aeneas was only a spectator, whereas *he* was taking part in the games. He was, however, younger than Aeneas and more of an athlete.

Marett has written (and the statement has often been made
by others, including many psycho-analytic writers) that
fears, though not all of one type, are of one parentage, the
father and mother of all fears being, biologically speaking,
the fear of death.[1] Anthropologists speak of a deep horror
of death as being universal among mankind. In Hastings'
Encyclopædia of Religion and Ethics (1911), an account of funeral
rites among peoples the world over is introduced thus :

" The horror of death is universal among mankind. It
depends not so much on the pain that often accompanies
dissolution as upon the mystery of it and the results to the
subject and to the survivors—the cessation of the old familiar
relations between them and the decomposition of the body.
This horror has given rise to an obstinate disbelief in the
necessity of death, and to attempts, continually repeated in
spite of invariable disastrous experience of failure, to escape
it. . . . The picture thus presented of the desperate refusal
of mankind to accept a cardinal condition of existence is
one of the most pathetic in the history of the race." (25).

It was formerly held that the savage feared death more
than the civilized do, but Hocart (28) states that, on the
contrary, the horror of death is greater in civilized man than
in the savage.

" Death customs are generally supposed to have their
roots in the emotions, especially dread. Savages, among
whom death customs are generally more elaborate than
among the highly civilized peoples, are alleged to feel an

---

[1] Bibliographical List, 49.i. From the viewpoint of psycho-analysis,
however, the matter is not undisputed. To Stekel's insistence on the
opinion that every fear is ultimately a fear of death, Freud has opposed
the point that " death is an abstract concept with a negative content for
which no unconscious correlative can be found " (*The Ego and the Id*).
Freud appears to place the fear of death (in any other sense than as
an immediately threatening external danger) as later in development
than the superego, and the superego as a resultant of the Œdipus
complex.

overwhelming fear of death, which prompts measures for self-protection. This is not confirmed by observation. Savages live and die publicly, so that the sight of death is often familiar from childhood. In the more civilized groups death is hidden. Contact with it is much rarer and for that reason gives a greater shock ; it is their greater horror of it that makes them keep it out of sight."

This characteristic of civilization—to keep the physical processes of death out of sight—is an ancient custom, but it is only within comparatively recent years that we have also been expected to keep death out of mind, and children have been shielded from the thought of it. The child of seventeenth-century Protestantism was early made familiar with ideas of Heaven and Hell. Bunyan's *Christian*

" brake his mind to his wife *and children ;* and thus he began to talk to them : O my dear Wife, said he, and you the children of my bowels. . . . I am for certain informed that this our City will be burned with fire from Heaven ; in which fearful overthrow, both myself, with thee my Wife, and you my sweet Babes, shall miserably come to ruine, except . . . some way of escape can be found."[1]

It was Dr. Samuel Johnson's earliest religious teaching, when he was a little child in bed with his mother, that Heaven was a place to which good people went, and Hell a place to which bad people went.[2] *The Pilgrim's Progress* was approved as sound reading-matter for children as well as adults, and many moral tales were produced for children's especial benefit. Dr. Johnson's earliest religious teaching was taken for granted as the common knowledge of all children.

---

[1] J. Bunyan, *The Pilgrim's Progress*, 1678. The book was translated into many languages within a few years, and has continued to sell ever since. Bunyan himself says, at the opening of the second part, how much it was being read in America.

[2] J. Boswell, *Life of Samuel Johnson*, 1791. Johnson was born in 1709.

" Does this child know the nature of an oath ? " said the Magistrate.

" You know where little boys go to that tell fibs ? " said the Police-Inspector. " Coorse you do ! Speak up, my lad. Where will you go to if you don't speak the truth ? Bein' on oath, mind you ! "[1]

The education commonly given to children in the mid-nineteenth century doubtless fully justified the policeman's confidence in little Joe's response, although Joe himself (aged seven) did not. He answered, " If I tells lies I shall go to Heaven because of the Divine Grace." His instruction had been unorthodox. But he obviously had not a doubt of the Inspector's meaning, and could have named the event which would be expected to intervene between heaven and the police-court.

In fact, the impression is often given that in these earlier times the child, so far from being shielded from the thought of death, had it thrust upon him. But in all such references it is notable that it is not simply the process of death, biologically considered, that is thrust upon the notice of the child ; it is the life after death, the conditions of immortality. The attitude is itself a defence against the fear of dissolution.

It is also characterized by the excessive affect of civilization. Undoubtedly the hope of conquering death by achieving personal immortality arose very early in the development of man.[2] But the after-life of savage imagination lays no such deep shadow across the life of this world as the Christian revelation did. In the after-life of savages

----

[1] W. de Morgan, *Joseph Vance*, 1906. The incident is supposed to occur in 1848 or '49. *Cf.* a somewhat similar scene with another Joe, in Dickens' *Bleak House*.

[2] " Instead of succumbing to a fear so everlasting in its enmity, man for many thousands of years has met it squarely with the aid of a no less everlasting hope. . . . He will be immortal ; he will overcome the time-process and see it out. Thus, then, so far as force of will could do it, Neanderthal man, to whom we grudge the name of Homo Sapiens, achieved a future life." (Marett. Bib. List, 49.ii.)

there is often a second death ; after that the departed spirit fades away to nothingness, and may be forgotten by those connected with him in his worldly life, if indeed their forgetfulness were not a condition necessary' for his complete annihilation.[1] But for Christians, the second death is traditionally preceded by a Day of Doom, when the fearful and unbelieving, with the wicked, are cast into a lake of fire.[2]

Hell is not a *savage* idea.

" Even when an implacable hell finds a place in a primitive mythology, no organized attempt is made to bring its horrors home to the imagination, and thereby to tyrannize over the soul, as among advanced peoples."[3]

Men who have pictured the Christian hell and the Last Judgment have possessed also the highest attributes of civilization, for Michael Angelo painted it on the wall of the Sistine Chapel.

With the advance of civilization, the hope and fear which combined to produce the primitive idea of immortality as a defence against death-anxiety split apart ; heaven separates from hell, and there are different terms of admission. Those who enter heaven abandon all fear (" And the gates of it—the City of Heaven—shall not be shut at all by day : and there shall be no night there ") ; those at the gate of hell abandon hope. The living participate in these projected experiences ; some gain eternity in imagination, unfettered by time ; others suffer hell on earth, as the poet Cowper did. It was to ensure their arrival in Heaven that children in former times were not spared accounts of Hell. When the mind is fixed on such dread alternatives, the physiological

[1] Many references to such a belief may be found in anthropological studies. See Frazer, Bib. List, 19.*a*.ii.

[2] The Bible. The Book of the Revelation of St. John the Divine, chs. xx, xxi.

[3] Marett, *op. cit.*, p. 51 (49.iii).

process of death appears as but an incident, transitory and unimportant ; merely the gateway of the after-life, and a new birth. Death is out of focus when the gaze is fixed on the life beyond it ; this is a motive for the high colouring of Heaven and Hell. Thus an impulse which formerly led adults to stress, to children, the thought of death as after-life, was the fear of death as physical process and immediate loss. The impulse which leads them to shield children from thoughts of death to-day is fundamentally the same, but the hope has been abandoned, and the fear displaced or repressed.

In the education of English children, between the fullness of Church teaching and the modern repression of thought of death, came an interval when adults seemed to enjoy watching the child play with the idea. He was no longer given moral tales and hymns, or forced to spend Sundays learning collects and catechism. But he was taught for recitation some " pretty piece," which treated the subject in a way more attractive to the age. Babies recited " We are Seven " or " Casabianca " until promoted to the junior school, when they intoned instead " The Burial of Sir John Moore at Corunna," " The Destruction of Sennacherib," or " Horatius " from *The Lays of Ancient Rome*. They were amused with the fate of the chubby lad Augustus, or Harriet and the matches (30). Lewis Carroll introduced the idea of death into the Postscript to the *Alice* books, with gentle seriousness :

" Surely your gladness need not be the less for the thought that you will one day see a brighter dawn than this. . . ."

There are no such postscripts to children's books to-day, and even Ruthless Rhymes and Cautionary Tales are out of date.

What is the effect of such different treatment by adults on the thoughts and attitudes of the children ? It is a question not easy to answer ; certainly not to be answered here. I can only suggest two considerations in connection with it.

The first is that religion, wherever it has a hold, performs a function. The cure is not, though to outsiders it may seem, worse than the disease. Religion offers relief from anxieties, even when it leads to suttee, martyrdom or sacrifice ; and not only relief to the survivors. "Though He slay me, yet will I trust in Him," has its reward both in life and in death. The Calvinist and the Catholic braved the hell they vividly imagined, through insistence on justification by faith and through grace ; underlying this theological doctrine is a deep understanding of the power of suggestion, the paralyzing nature of anxiety, and the childish (or unconscious) tendency to assume too much moral responsibility. This insistence determines that hope shall tip the scale, as far as the self is concerned. The attainment of heaven was never in any Christian doctrine made absolutely dependent on *works*, the outward-showing morality. But apparent goodness gave further assurance of inward grace. Agnosticism about the after-life, if it becomes a creed, does so by offering some form of mental exercise for the toleration of anxieties.[1] Often the agnostic also strives to secure all the survival he believes possible by producing children who will not forget him, or immortal works. Milton, rejecting it as un-Christian, felt this desire for fame to be " the last infirmity of noble minds."

[1] A modern expression of agnosticism as a creed, offering a mental exercise for the toleration of anxieties, is the following :

" Freethought is knowledge of the relation of the finite to the infinite . . . it is an extremely difficult, if not impossible, task to be a free-thinker. I cannot deny it. It is extremely difficult to approach closely any religious ideal. . . . The relief of spiritual misery . . . is the mission of free thought. . . . In the discovery of new truth . . . we find its noblest function, its deepest meaning. Not by myth, not by guesses of the imagination is the problem of life to be solved ; but by earnest application, by downright hard work of the brain, spread over the life-time of many men, extending even to the life-time of the world ; for the solution of the problem is identical with the mental development of humanity, and none can say where that shall end." (Karl Pearson, *The Ethic of Freethought*.)

These attitudes of the agnostic find expression in the final paragraph of Tacitus' *Agricola* :

" Si quis piorum manibus locus, si, ut sapientibus placet, non cum corpore extinguuntur magnae animae, placide quiescas, nosque, domum tuam, ab infirmo desiderio et muliebribus lamentis ad contemplationem virtutum tuarum voces, quas neque lugeri neque plangi fas est. Admiratione te potius quam temporalibus laudibus, et, si natura suppeditet, aemulatione decoremus. . . . Id filiae quoque uxorique praeceperim, sic patris, sic mariti memoriam venerari, ut omnia facta dictaque eius secum revolvant, formamque ac figuram animi magis quam corporis complectantur ; non quia intercedendum putem imaginibus, quae marmore aut aere finguntur ; sed ut vultus hominum, ita simulacra vultus imbecilia ac mortalia sunt, forma mentis aeterna, quam tenere et exprimere non per alienam materiam et artem, sed tuis ipse moribus possis. Quicquid ex Agricola amavimus, quicquid mirati sumus, manet mansurumque est in animis hominum, in aeternitate temporum, fama rerum. Nam multos veterum velut inglorios et ignobiles oblivio obruit ; Agricola posteritati narratus et traditus superstes erit."

(If there be any habitation for the spirits of good men ; if, as the wise are pleased to believe, great souls do not perish with the body, thou mayest calmly rest, and call us of thine own home from weak longing and feminine laments to the contemplation of thy virtue, which it is not right we should grieve over or bewail. Let us honour thee with admiration rather than with passing praises, and with emulation, if our natures make that possible. . . . This foremost I would suggest to thy daughter and thy wife, that they should honour the memory of their father and husband as though revolving within their minds all his deeds and words, and embracing rather the form and shape of his soul than of his body. Not that I consider that images formed in marble or bronze should be forbidden ; but as the features of men, and representations of their features, are alike without significance and perishable, while the form of the mind is eternal, thou canst retain and express it not through an alien material and art, but through thy behaviour itself. Whatever in Agricola we have loved, whatever we have admired, remains and will remain in men's minds, through the eternity of time, by the recounting of events. For oblivion has overwhelmed many of the men of old among the inglorious and ignoble ; but Agricola, whose life has been told and handed down to posterity, will yet survive.)

Every form of religion, in the sight of its adherents, offers more, in the relief of distress about the ending of the individual life, than it takes away in hope and blind security. Any form of religion sincerely held by the adults of a group to which a child belongs, may provide that child with an " escape into reality," when he spontaneously turns to it. Such escapes are often valuable and sometimes critical and essential stages in the child's mental adjustment.

The second consideration is that *any* religion may be used sadistically to suggest or add to children's fears, instead of to allay them. This is the more obvious, the more positive the tenets of the religion are ; that is to say, the more the hope and fear on which all religion is based, are dissociated and projected. But the agnostic attitude is to many children quite intolerable ; infants may respond with passionate anger or misery if answered " I don't know " by an adult on any matter in which they feel concern. No form of religion is proof against cruel application to children ; any, unsuitably presented either in words or example, may fail to give the individual child the relief from anxiety which he seeks. In this connection the term *religion* is considered synonymous with the integration in each individual of his attitude to death.

CHAPTER V

FASCINATED by the exploration of the gloomy depths of the mind, we may overlook what is lying on the surface. Anxious not to refuse recognition to the children's impulses to kill their mothers, fathers, brothers, and other dear ones, we may omit to find out what the word *dead* means to them when they direct their thoughts consciously to its meaning.

In order to collect such information, we must ensure that the word is insulated from incidental emotional charges for each individual child.

With this aim in view, the word *dead* was added to the Vocabulary List of the Revised (1937) Stanford-Binet Intelligence Scale, as already described in Chapter II, and 91 children were asked for a definition of its meaning in the course of administration of the whole scale.

NEGATIVE RESULTS

Six children proved unable to give any response. Four of these were suffering from a general " nervousness " which inhibited verbal responses over the test as a whole. With two children the inhibition of response had reference to the word *dead* only.

CLASSIFICATION OF RESPONSES

The remaining 85 responses were examined with regard to the character of the meaning they presented, and classified

G   81

on the ground of differences in this character, in five categories (or more roughly three, with subdivisions in the upper and the lower categories). Verbal facility, rapidity of response, rationality, comprehension, exactitude or elaboration of meaning, were all discounted, in favour of the character-type of the meaning given by the child verbally as the primary one, in his response.

When there was doubt whether the child *was* incapable of expressing a concept of death verbally (but only then), evidence obtained from other responses was taken into account. For example, when Henry F. answered (during the Vocabulary Test) " I think I don't know dead," but in a later context said of a little dog (of whom it had been mentioned that he had died), " 'E died. 'Cos the dog ate too much bones "—he was judged to have some conception of death, although a limited one.

The categories were then named, A to E, in an order corresponding to the degree of understanding they appeared to show ; A being apparent ignorance. The age-distribution of the children in each category was noted, and the numbers of subjects falling in each category at each year of age, in respect of both chronological and mental age.

(Two responses remained outside the categories. A child of five years replied simply " dyin'," and another of 9 : 11 gave a frown, looked puzzled, and said " died.")

DESCRIPTION OF DEFINITIONS ACCORDING TO CATEGORIES

A. The child expresses ignorance of the meaning of the word, or fails to respond.

B. There is evidence of some meaning being attached to the word. The meaning is limited. There is no explicit association of the meaning with a functioning subject in the response itself. Ignorance may be expressed.

Examples : " adn't 'ad no dinner "
            " to go asleep "

C. The child shows by his response that he is sure he understands the concept ; there is application to human beings, and frequently further elaborations which refer to aspects of death not logically or biologically essential.

Examples : " somebody's dead "
" when people's dead "
" somebody dies, and they have a funeral "
" when you're in your coffin and you're layin' in it "

D. Transitional between C and E. Reference to humanity exclusively, may be combined with reference to logical or biological essentials, but there is insufficient generalization either of the logical or biological aspect to warrant classification in Class E.

Examples : " when a person doesn't live any more "
" when you're dead, m'm, you can't come alive again, madam "

E. Reference is made to logical or biological essentials.

Examples : " not living "
" when you have no pulse and no temperature and can't breathe "

THE RELATION OF THE CATEGORIES (A–E) WITH AGE

The tables given below show the relation between these categories and (a) the children's age in years (b) their *mental age* as given by the Intelligence Test.[1] These tables

---

[1] The material does not provide suitable data for the computation of a correlation coefficient. The intelligence distribution in the sample was not normal (see p. 28 ff.). The totals in many of the cells are so small as to make the method of mean-square-contingency unreliable. The product-moment formula is not applicable because one of the characters is categoric. The cases in columns 12–, 13– in the C.A. table were recruited on a different basis from the main body, because the Story-Completion Test was not considered suitable for children of normal intelligence at these ages.

A correlation ratio was, however, computed for both tables, after rejection of all these 12+ cases of the C.A. table from both tables, and

show that there is a correspondence between increase in age and the changes indicated by the categories A–E, and they suggest that intelligence (as measured by this scale)

TABLE II
The Relation between Chronological Age and " Dead " Definition

	-5	5-	6-	7-	8-	9-	10-	11-	12-	13-	TOTAL
E ..				1	1	3	2				7
D ..				1	1	3	1			1	7
C ..		6	6	14	6	8	5	5	3	3	56
B ..	3	3	1	1						1	9
A ..	1	1	1			1					4
TOTAL	4	10	8	14	9	11	11	8	3	5	83

TABLE III
The Relation between Mental Age and " Dead " Definition

	-5	5-	6-	7-	8-	9-	10-	11-	12-	13-	TOTAL
E ..					1	2	1	1		2	7
D ..				1	2	3	1				7
C ..	1	2	15	13	9	5	6	3	2		56
B ..	1	5	3								9
A ..	3	1									4
TOTAL	5	8	18	13	10	8	11	5	3	2	83

grouping together of all cases under age 6 : 0 (C.A. and M.A.), and above age 11 : 0 (M.A.), so as to reduce the number of columns and increase the cell totals. The total population used was then 75.

These correlation ratios were found to be :

Chronological Age with Response-category .. 0.59 (η)
Mental Age with Response-category .. .. 0.66 (η)

The correlation between C.A. and M.A. after rejection of the same (12+) cases was found by product-moment formula to be 0.67 (r). In a population where intelligence is normally distributed this correlation might be expected to be higher.

TABLE IV

The Relation between Chronological and Mental Age of Subjects for "Dead" Definitions

M.A.	C.A. −5	5−	6−	7−	8−	9−	10−	11−	12−	13−.	TOTAL (M.A.)
13 up							1	1			2
12−								1	1	1	3
11−						1	1	1	1	1	5
10−						2	6	1	1	1	11
9−					1	3	2	1		1	8
8−		2		2	2	2	1	1			10
7−			1	5	3	1		2		1	13
6−		4	4	6	2	2					18
5−	2	3	2		1						8
to−5	2	1	1	1							5
TOTAL (C.A.)	4	10	8	14	9	11	11	8	3	5	83

may be a factor in furthering such changes, possibly of even greater weight than accidental experience.

The chance of any child having relevant accidental experience of death may be supposed to increase in constant ratio to chronological age, when a sufficiently large number of cases is taken. The development of the change in type of response, however, varies somewhat more closely with mental age than with chronological age (though the difference is scarcely enough to be considered significant). This suggests that an innate factor is no less weighty than specific stimuli in the environment.[1]

It is clear from the tables that the year 7–8 is critical in the development of the concept of death according to these categories. The way in which the main change turns graphically around this age is indeed very striking, particularly in the mental-age table. No child whose mental age was over 7 : 0 gave a response below C category ; every child of mental age 7–8 (and every child of this chronological age) gave an answer in this category ; no child whose mental age was under 8 : 0 gave a response of D or E category.

This perfect symmetry is undoubtedly partly due to chance and it also owes something to the coarseness of the grouping. The age-gap between the A–B and the D–E categories is actually more than a year ; it is over two years. The highest mental age in B class is 6 : 7 ; the lowest in D class is 8 : 9. But when allowance is made for both these factors, the significance of the eighth year is still remarkable.

This numerical result confirms strikingly the relation between age and certain stages of mental development

[1]Evidence from two individual cases, however, suggested that specific objective experience is by no means negligible in determining the category into which a child's response will fall. Two of the dullest children tested had had recent experience of a father's death, and each falls at the lowest limit of his category, reckoned by mental age. That is to say, through excessively " favourable " experience these children have scraped into a category to which their mental abilities would probably not otherwise have brought them.

indicated by Professor Piaget. In his work, *The Child's Conception of Causality*, he writes :

In the course of our studies on child psychology we had expected to fix upon 7–8 as the age before which no genuinely physical explanation could be given of natural phenomena. Our present enquiry entirely confirms this expectation. After 7–8 the more positive forms of causality gradually supplant the others, and we can say that at the age of about 11–12 the evolution is completed. There is, therefore . . . a process of evolution (such that the child proceeds from) confusion of the self and the universe (to) progressive separation with objectification of the causal sequences. (53.*b*.iii).

The present data bear out Professor Piaget's findings as to the significance of the year 7–8 as the turning-point in development, and the progressive objectification of the child's attitude to phenomena.   The difference between the responses in C category and those in D–E categories is largely one of objectivity, although other factors are also involved in the total change of attitude.

Piaget's further finding, that the evolution towards objectivity proceeds from a state of mind when the self and the universe are confused, also, in a modified form, receives some support from the present material. Here the relevant data is to be found in the A–B responses, as contrasted with those of C category.

It is one of the main distinctions between A–B and C categories, that in the C responses the idea of *dead* has specific reference to humanity. It may appear strange that such a change should correlate with an advance in mental age, since death is *not* peculiar to humanity, and the greater particularity of the application is logically an error. Yet from observation of a number of cases the experimenter was left in no doubt that it is the earlier form of definition, apparently more general, which is psychologically more limited.

To give instances : Daphne S., aged 4 : 8, with a mental age of 3 : 11, defined *dead* as *it don't go on*. This followed definitions of *orange* as *orange . . . orange . . . apple*, and of *straw* as *drink out of*. When Daphne was shown a picture of a group of men reading a newspaper, she said, " I'm going to read some papers," and to a picture of adults in a canoe, " I'm going into the boat." Chloe O., aged 5 : 5, with a mental age of 5 : 0, defined *dead* as *to go asleep*. In order to make a test of the extent of her understanding of the word she was later asked the following problem : " What is silly about this : ' A little girl had a dog, but he died last year. He was two years old then, so now he's three.' " Although the problem, as such, was beyond Chloe's powers of comprehension, it had its effect, for in the Story-Completion Test, when asked why the little girl was sorry, she answered :

(Chloe :) Abou' t' li'l doggie.
E. : Why was she sorry about the little doggie ?
Chloe (after a considerable pause) : Because . . . because 'e was in 'ospital.

The definitions given by Daphne and Chloe appear on the face of them to be objective and impersonal. But the objectivity evidently has quite a different psychological foundation from that of the D–E categories.

In connection with children's definitions in general, Terman has remarked on impersonal forms which are immature. He points out that the functional type of definition commonly given by young children shows two grammatical forms which correlate significantly with mental age. The use of the infinitive and impersonal is earlier. The younger child will say, when asked what we mean by *chair*, " to sit on," while a child of somewhat higher mental age will respond, " you sit on it." In this latter definition, *people* are definitely referred to ; in the former, no distinction is made between humanity and the world in general (69.i).

The definition " to go asleep " corresponds with " to sit on," and the definition " someone's dead," which sounds comparatively so inept, corresponds with the more advanced form for chair : " you sit on it."

The *general* nature of this psychological development is shown by the fact that death is *not correctly* made specific to human beings. The process affects the concept of death merely as it affects all conceptual thought. Humanity, people, have begun to stand out as a figure-character from the background of the universe. The relation of any object to people is one of its most striking attributes at this age.

In contrast, the early, impersonal (but still functional) definitions show confusion of thought. There is a lack of analysis of the world of phenomena. It is as though, in the young child's world at this stage (A–B category) where things are considered in terms of function, three kinds of functioning are cognized. These three are, firstly, the perceptual self (ego), doing and suffering, clearly distinguished from the rest of the universe ; secondly, the fantasy self, as victim and as omnipotence strangely inextricable from the universe ; and thirdly, as main determinant of things and events of life, a great mass of happenings, *goings-on, doings,* in the background, in which adults mingle with impersonal impulses (such as *time for dinner*) in the causation of events, and which (unless the child's omnipotent self becomes specifically concerned in some part of it) proceeds by some unanalyzed and inevitable force of circumstance. Amid this mass of happenings, the only clearly cognized relationships are the relationships to himself ; *in so far as his world is explicable, expressible,* it is thus *egocentric* (in Professor Piaget's terminology). But the expressible world of the child is only a very small part of his whole mental universe.

This, I would suggest, is roughly the psychological background of the stage represented by A–B category and the Terman infinitive-functional definitions. When the child reaches the stage represented by C category and the *you* or *someone* definitions, he has left this earlier attitude behind and has begun to distinguish *people* as functional (doing and suffering) ; that is to say, the general *goings-on* in the background have had distinction made as between personal and impersonal forces. Further, the personal forces connected with these general happenings have been to some extent identified with (or rather, seen as analogous to) the perceptual self (the ego). The area in which the omnipotent self can functionally mingle has become proportionately reduced.

Thus in a sense we may say that there is progressively less confusion of the self with the universe in the child's mind, and that this evolution is illustrated by the changes in definitions of *dead* at different mental ages ; but we should not consider that there was evidence at any stage of the child's life for his confusion of self and universe in any completeness (nor indeed for a complete *distinction* between the two by the adult). We believe that there is, in fact, evidence for the child's making distinction between self and universe at a very early age in his perceptual experience. This question will be discussed more fully in the next chapter.

In studying the development in children of one idea in particular, one is necessarily led to compare the findings with the theories of Professor Piaget, because his work on the development of childish thought in general is so outstanding. That work also has certain interesting observations to offer in connection with our main subject. Piaget has suggested that there may exist a close relation between the development of the idea of death and intellectual development in general. In the study of questions spontaneously asked by a boy of 6–7 (Del), preoccupation with this idea was particularly noticed (53.*a*). Piaget believes that this interest is of importance in connection with the development of the idea of chance. He maintains that it is a major distinction between child and adult thought, that the child does not allow its share to chance in the nexus of events ; he (the child) tries to find a reason for everything, including many things which the adult will accept as fortuitous (that is to say, resulting from *statistical causality*).

Piaget traces the psychological process behind the conflict which makes death such an interest and problem for the child. At this stage, he says, the idea of the fortuitous does not exist ; causality presupposes a " maker "—God, the parents, etc., and the questions refer to the intentions they may have had.

" If the child at this stage is puzzled by the problem of death, it is precisely because in his conception of things death is inexplicable. . . . Death is the fortuitous and mysterious phenomenon *par excellence.* And in the questions about plants, and animals, and the human body, it is those which refer to death which will cause the child to leave behind him the stage of pure finalism, and to acquire the notion of statistical causality or chance." (53.*a*. ii ; also see 53.*b* and *c*.)

To the small child, according to Piaget, causation is equivalent to psychological motivation or anthropomorphic activity. God or man makes things ; that is how they come ; that, for instance, is how the mountains around Geneva come to be how and where they are. God or man intends things, that is why they happen. This view of causality is closely bound up with the belief in the omnipotence of thought and wish, through that characteristic of childhood which Piaget has described in detail under the name of egocentricity, and has shown to have affinity with the characteristic which Freud has named narcissism (53.*b*.i).

If the idea of death has special importance for intellectual development at this stage, it must be because it presents itself as proof of the ultimate impotence of thought and desire. Death comes despite the wish of the sufferer and the desires of those *who love* the dead. It is inevitable and comes to all. It proves to the imaginary-omnipotent that he is not omnipotent ; but it only does so if love is dominant in the emotion aroused by the (imagined or real) victim.   If in that emotion-complex, which is necessarily ambivalent, the hate-aspect has not been effectively repressed, the logic may start from other premises and follow other lines, which have been already indicated on page 59. A sense of guilt appears, while the sense of omnipotence is not abandoned. Individual omnipotence is inconsistent with causality based on scientific deduction.   It is therefore highly symbolic of the mental development that underlies all conscious logic, that the study of logic traditionally opens with the statement that *All men are Mortal.*

Piaget traces the earlier attitude of psychological motiva-tion as cause, to the emotional life of the child in the cradle, where the psycho-analyst also finds the source of later mental attitudes. The child's thoughts about death therefore form a link, in Piaget's genetic scheme, between the emotional life of the earliest period, and the intellectual developments which follow the stage that he entitles *egocentric.* He has been accused by Dr. Susan Isaacs of providing no such link within the inner psychological life of the child (33.*a*). It must be admitted that he himself has not stressed the idea of death as such a link, and has only lightly in passing suggested it as such.

Without further reference to theory based on other researches, let us examine in more detail the responses which fall into C category ; that is to say, the large majority of all the definitions, representing the central group in age, hinging on the eighth year, and completely cutting off the infantile from the " mature " groups.

It is evident that between two periods of childhood when the meaning of death is different, there occurs a period of elaboration of the idea. This begins generally at mental age 6–7, though occasionally earlier, and is generally concluded by (and often before) mental age 13. A seven-year-old will probably be passing through this stage. He may not have reached it till about 6 : 6 ; he may leave it by M.A. 9 : 0 ; it will probably last two years, maybe longer.

The essential characteristics of the death definitions of this period have already been mentioned. The idea has become a familiar one, without taking any very definite objective shape. The realization that human beings die overshadows the greater generality of death as a biological fact. Special aspects fill in the picture ; positive aspects, primarily of emotional significance : funerals, coffins, ambulances, murderers, lying down flat, etc. Death is thought of in terms of human experience. To think of it as biological process, or as negation of life, is a distinctly later stage, with a transitional stage in between.

The impression made by the C responses as a whole is that they represent a fantasy-phase of thought. The idea of death is being autistically assimilated. Anxieties about it are being worked over. What the child attends to, in objective phenomena, are those things which symbolize unconscious concepts connected with his conscious concepts of death. These are the very things which men have produced culturally for the same purpose, to relieve anxieties about death. To the child at this stage, death is not essentially an objective, biological phenomenon in its own right. He has so far accepted reality as to assimilate a general fact ; people die. That has taken him out of stage B. But the fact does not attract him ; he does not look straight at it ; he looks round it. He looks at the appurtenances of it ; he fantasies causes for it. Coffins, burial rites, the primitive idea that there must have been ill-will, a murderer—these are typical elaborations of the child of C category when he defines death.[1]

[1] One must hesitate before drawing too easy conclusions about the intellectual development which is actually taking place during a certain

The essential meaning given in the response is far from being its only interesting and significant characteristic. We can modify some words of Terman and say that our purpose is not only to find what meaning the child gives the word he is asked to define, but to find how he apperceives the word, or the object for which it stands. How he apperceives death often becomes apparent from the context of the definition. Among the younger children we have already mentioned the responses of Daphne ("it don't go on"), Chloe ("to go asleep") and Henry ("it died 'cos it ate too much bones").

Chloe also equated death with going to hospital. This equation is commonly found in children of A and B categories and occurs occasionally also in C category in conjunction with fuller comprehension. Among children of a mental age of five years it sometimes seems to be a complete equation; they may attach no other meaning to the idea of death. For instance, Joan U. (C.A. 6 : 9 ; M.A. 5 : 2) defines *dead* as "send it in 'ospital." Later, when looking at a picture of a gun, she is asked what people do with it and answers, "Shoot." Asked what happens to people who are shot she replies, "Go in 'ospital"; an answer reasonable enough, but adding something nevertheless in confirmation of the equation. And when presented with the little-dog absurdity (see p. 88) she said, "The little girl was silly." "Why?" "'Cos she made the dog ill."

period from the responses produced at that age. Such responses (unless the stimulus question has been put with educational intent and has educational results) will not at all stages normally represent the highest achievements of the child's intellect in regard to the problem. For one thing, the main preoccupation may be with fantasy-aspects of the problem; for another thing, there will be a time-lag; *habits* of thought will play a part in determining the reply. Thought on any one subject has its "scatter" in the mind. The reply will probably come from near the mean of the distribution; but the intellectual work is being done (to mix the metaphor) on the upper levels.

Everything here points to an equation of the idea of illness—hospital treatment—death.

In the same wholesale way, below the mentality represented by C category, the idea of death may be equated with deprivation of food, as by Alfred R., aged 6 : 6 (M.A. 5 : 8) who said *dead* meant " 'adn't 'ad no dinner."[1]

Of the 56 definitions in C category, 28 lacked all elaboration ; that is to say, the child responded with " somebody's dead," or some similarly brief and repetitive reply.

When any elaboration of this simple theme occurred the commonest reference was to *burial*. Eleven children referred to a grave, a coffin, or the burial process. Next on the list in order of frequency comes the context of *aggression ;* death is seen as the outcome of an attack. Irene K. (5 : 3) defines *dead* as *somebody's killed.* Margaret E. (7 : 8) pauses, purses her mouth in a way habitual with her, and physically symbolic of repression, and replies *somebody what's been killed.* Joe Y., aged 12 : 7 (M.A. 6 : 6 ; mentally defective), goes so far as to define *dead* as *when people get murdered.* Two more children also gave answers in this sub-group. Three children in C category elaborated with *illness* or *hospital* references. In addition to these there are references to *heaven, sleep,* the *prone position, inability to be active* in some way, and to details of *dissolution.*   .

The references to *heaven* were only two ; they occurred at almost opposite ends of the age range : Rose E., a friendly, plump little girl with a great sense of humour and of her own dignity (C.A. 5 : 9, M.A. 7 : 2) answered, " Sometimes you're dead," with a laugh. (E. : And what then ?) " Then you go in 'eaven, if you're good." Hilda Y., a mental-

---

[1] In America, however, children apparently equate death with over-feeding rather than under-feeding. This, at least, is how the nutrition problem appears in Schilder and Wechsler's study of *Children's Attitudes to Death* (58). In England, such a possibility only occurred to one subject of research—Henry, already quoted—and the victim was in this case a dog.

defective aged 14 : 6, said *dead* was " like when they're dead." (E. : And then ?) " Then they go to heaven."

With several children the primary elaboration of *dead* was *the prone position*. Fred M., for instance, defines it as " when you're in your coffin and you're layin' in it," and he waves his hand horizontally. Joanna F., 5 : 8, responds, " Someone's dead, and I'll show you how to be dead. Shall I draw a person dead ? (She quickly picks up a pencil and draws a rough little figure of someone lying down.) Shall I do a person alive ? " (She then draws a figure standing up.) Betty H.'s definition (her age is 9 : 0) is, " When somebody's lying unc . . . unconsciously." Pamela Q. (a clinic case, aged 10 : 11) said, " When you're in your coffin. When you don't know where you are."

Some of these involve with the idea of the prone position, a more definite idea of *impotence*. Only one child brought out that idea explicitly : Irene T., 7 : 10, said " dead "— " means somebody's dead and they can't do anything."

The response of Alfred I. (8 : 2) was a rather unusual one ; in fact among these subjects it was unique :

E. : Dead ? Alfred : When you die.
E. : And then ? Alfred : All the beetles eat your eyes out.
(E. apparently showed some uncertainty whether she had heard aright the word " beetles.") Alfred : . . . Insects.

THE INFLUENCE OF HOME TEACHING ON CHILDREN'S DEFINITIONS OF DEATH

In collecting the data no attempt was made to deal with the factor of home education (religious or other) in the children's ideas of death. Incidents occurred, however, to show that the influence of this factor on the placing of responses in the five categories was probably negligible. The most intelligent of all the children tested was Sheila B., aged 5 : 7, with a mental age of 8 : 3 on Stanford-Binet (I.Q. 148).

Her definition of " dead " fell into the C category : " When people get dead." (Q.: What happens then?) " They go in their grave."

Sheila's elder brother, Patrick, was aged 8 : 10 ; S-B mental age, 11 : 11, I.Q. 135. (He had recently won second place in a scholarship examination.) His response fell into E category : " A body that has no life in it." The eldest child, Marian, aged 10 : 9 (S-B M.A. 14 : 6, I.Q. 135), also gave an answer in E category : " When you have no pulse and no temperature and can't breathe." (Since this testing, Marian has won a secondary school scholarship, although she has recently had diphtheria.)

These children came of an Irish Catholic family. The father was a foreman dock labourer—undoubtedly also a highly intelligent man, for Marian asked him in the dinner-hour some of the vocabulary list she had not known (at the level of Superior Adult II) and came back and gave his (correct) answers. Marian was at this date taking the part of the Virgin Mary in the school nativity play. These three children, from the same home and certainly not taught any religious scepticism (one of Patrick's wishes was to go to heaven when he died), gave different responses, all in accordance with their mental age.

The same appears with Henry F. and his sister Josie. Their respective ages were 5 : 2 (M.A. 6 : 2, I.Q. 119) and 7 : 0 (M.A. 7 : 6, I.Q. 107). Henry says, " I think I don't know dead," but later suggests that the death of a dog was " 'cos the dog ate too much bones, 'e died. " (Q.: After that?) "They took 'im to a grave." His response falls into Class B. Josie answers :

When somebody's layin' dead . . . they was dead, you see. There was a large grave there. Somebody said some-body died down there. I think she was ever so old. We saw Mr. Maguire. . . ."

—the whole story referring to an actual death which occurred
H

during the hop-picking on which the family was engaged in the previous summer holidays. This response falls into Class C. Then there is Desmond I., 9 : 6 (M.A. 10 : 3, I.Q. 108), and his brother Leslie, 11 : 0 (M.A. 10 : 6), country boys. Leslie's response comes in Class E, and Desmond's in Class C. (L. : "When you stop breathing and you don't move any more." D. : "Somebody who's dead.")

Without attempting to investigate the amount or kind of home teaching in any individual case, we therefore have some evidence for the view that it does not affect *the category* into which the child's response will fall.

Summary of Chapter V

1. When 91 children aged 3–13 were asked to give the meaning of *dead* in the course of a vocabulary list, the 83 responses available fell into five categories which had a significant correlation with both chronological and mental age ($\eta = 0.59$ and 0.66 respectively).

2. The majority of the responses (56) fell into the median category C. All the children of age 7–8 gave answers in this category. No children under 8 : 0 gave answers above C category. No children over mental age 7 : 0 gave answers below C category.

3. Responses below C category showed either ignorance or markedly limited conceptions of *dead*, and the latter were occasionally expressed impersonally. C responses were marked by application to humanity and by elaboration of cultural-symbolic aspects of death. Above C category responses tended to be objective, logical or biological.

4. Parallels were traced between the evolution of the conception of *dead* as shown by the categories, and Piaget's hypotheses of the psychological development of the child. The age-levels he gives for an evolution of conceptual thought towards objectivity were confirmed. It was considered to what extent the impersonality of some of the B definitions indicated an origin of this evolution in

confusion of self and universe. In connection also with Piaget's suggestion that the idea of death has particular importance for the development of the idea of the fortuitous, it was mooted that the logic of consciousness depends for its primacy on the idea of death only when that is combined with a dominance of love in the prevailing emotional attitude.

5. Responses in C category were analyzed to illustrate their cultural-symbolic trends.

6. Evidence was given to show that the categories were independent of religious teaching in the home.

CHAPTER VI

" I knew not that Men were born or should die "
Traherne.

RECORDS taken by relatives at home tend to suffer from
defects that Child Psychology has long recognized : they
have been summed up under the term *anecdotalism*. But it is
unlikely that a full science of early childhood can ever be
built up without using the observations of those with whom
the child is most intimate made in the environment to which
he is accustomed. So far from neglecting this type of evidence
in the present research, I have sought to collect as much
of it as possible under certain conditions whereby its validity
was, so far as might be, safeguarded. These conditions have
been already described in Chapter II. It cannot be claimed
that *anecdotalism* was always avoided in the material collected;
but if an anecdote has here and there been admitted, it
refers always to a child whose immediate reactions are also
being recorded, and is given not for its own sake but to enrich
the psychological context of the immediate observation.

This kind of material has another disadvantage : it cannot
easily be treated quantitatively. With the present records
quantitative treatment is out of the question. To bring
them into order for presentation they have been used to
illustrate certain theses. First have been placed those
propositions which appear to range themselves in a developmental sequence, and later, others which seem to possess an
outstanding general importance in the child's psychological
development. The data are presented quite separately from

the propositions, and obviously might be otherwise combined to present other theses. In illustrating genetic sequence by the home records, the categories described in the previous chapter have been kept in mind, and certain parallels appear. Where such parallels are found, chronological ages rarely correspond. Whether because of the comparatively high intelligence of the home-record children, or because of the fact that we are dealing with spontaneous activity in an intimate environment, the characteristic stages will be found to occur much earlier among the children observed at home.[1]

The propositions were suggested by the data which is presented under each head. When, in any case, other records collected by well-accredited psychological observers were found to have a bearing on the proposition, they also have been presented, after the newly collected material. The home-records of Rasmussen, Sully and the Katz parents, and the Malting House School records of Susan Isaacs have been used in this way. On the theoretical side the work of Piaget and of Freud, with their wealth of illustration, have been constantly kept in mind.

The children's pseudonyms in age order
Catherine Holland
Margaret Sage
Benedict Clement
Susanna Holland
Judith Anson
Jeremy Sage
Richard Clement
Francis Holland
Stephen Holme
Timothy Anson
Edward Holme.
Younger brothers : Anthony Sage, John Holland.

[1] Such discrepancies have been frequently noted, and psychologists have usually attributed them to the partiality of parents. Valentine has recently queried the soundness of this view. (*B.J.Ed.P.*, vii, 3, 1938.)

I.—*There is a stage in the child's development which is often not
passed through until speech is fairly well advanced, when the
child has no idea of death at all.*[1]

EXAMPLES.   (*a*) *Home Records.*

(i) *Ben, 3 : 2 (recorded after a considerable interval).*

F.[2] was cutting the hedge, assisted by Ben. Ben asked
why we had no dog. F. said that we had one once, before
Ben was born, but it was dead. Ben asked what happened
to it, and why we had none now. F. tried to explain. Ben
was puzzled and went into the house to M. and earnestly
attempted to express what he had been told (having meanwhile forgotten the words *dead* or *death*) so as to get his
mother to explain it to him.

(ii) *Stephen and Edward Holme, aged 4 : 10 and 2 : 5 (extract
from a letter from their mother when the record was begun).*

With regard to the concept of death. . . . Edward, of
course, hasn't appreciated it yet, but Stephen quite
frequently comes up against it and puzzles for a few minutes.
. . . The dead birds in poultry shops obviously puzzle him,
and at first he thought they were asleep.

EXAMPLES.   (*b*) *From other subjects of this research.*

In an infants' school where subjects were being tested,
there was a child aged 3 : 3, of whom the teacher reported
this incident : about four months previously she was alone
with her mother at home, when the mother, as she was
making a bed, suddenly fell upon the floor and apparently
died instantaneously of heart failure. The father returned to

---

[1] It is necessary to begin with a generalization which, being about a
negative condition, is difficult to illustrate satisfactorily and conclusively.
A child rarely asks the meaning of a word or phenomenon unless he
already has some interest in it, and the interest in itself implies some
degree of cognitive experience of the object. The examples given have
each some imperfection, and if they persuade of the truth of the proposition it must be cumulatively.

[2] " F." and " M." refer to the father and mother of the child of whom
the record is given in each case.

find the mother dead, and the little girl asleep on the floor beside her. These three formed the whole family, so that next day the father asked the headmistress to take the child in the school, although she was then below school age, as there was no one to look after her at home, and this was done. The class mistress reports this, and adds that the little girl, Marlene, said to her quite happily when she came to school, about the event: "Mother lay down on the floor and went to sleep, so I went to sleep, too."

The experimenter tested this child. Her mental age was only 2 : 8 (I.Q. 82). It was not possible to get further material about the development of her concept of death. The teacher reported her as an independent-minded child, always happy to do things for herself whenever she could.

EXAMPLES.   (c) *From published literature.*

Rasmussen reports the following incident of his daughter *Ruth, when just two years old;* the deduction from it in its context would, I think, most naturally be that Ruth had no actual conception of the meaning of the words she was using, but had got so far as to attach to " dead " the motor concomitants of sorrow :

"R., just two, made herself noticed by repeating the speech ' Pip is dead ' (Pip was the name given to a little girl she knew). This amused her for several days, and she said the words with the deepest pathos like a wailing woman. She lowered her head, drew up her eyebrows, half closed her eyes, and spoke with a lugubrious, subdued voice." (55.*a.*i).

The following is from a home record kept by a parent of a Malting House School child and published by *Dr. Susan Isaacs* in her records of the school :

" *Ursula, aged 3 : 4*
Ursula and her mother found a dead moth in the garden and discovered that it could not move. *Ursula :* Like the crab at St. Leonards and there was a boy took the pail and

got water and put it in to see if it would move and it didn't move. Why didn't it move, Mummie?" (33.*a*.ii).

A well-known passage in Traherne's *Centuries of Meditations*, written in the seventeenth century, gives an account of this stage of childish development through introspective reminiscence. The language is embroidered, but the thought bears the mark of sincerity and originality :

"All appeared new, and strange at first, inexpressibly rare and delightful and beautiful. . . . I knew not that there were any sins, or complaints or laws. . . . Everything was at rest, free and immortal. I knew nothing of sickness or death or rents or exaction, either for tribute or bread. . . . All Time was Eternity, and a perpetual Sabbath. . . .
The corn was orient and immortal wheat, which never should be reaped, nor was ever sown. I thought it had stood from everlasting to everlasting. . . . I knew not that (men) were born or should die ; but all things abided eternally in their proper places. Eternity was manifest in the light of Day, and something infinite behind everything appeared : which talked with my expectation and moved my desire. The city seemed to stand in Eden, or to be built in Heaven. The streets were mine, the temple was mine, the people were mine, their clothes and gold and silver were mine, as much as their sparkling eyes, fair skins and ruddy faces. The skies were mine, and so were the sun and moon and stars, and all the World was mine ; and I the only spectator and enjoyer of it. I knew no churlish proprieties (*i.e., property, possessions*), nor bounds nor divisions ; but all proprieties and divisions were mine, all treasures and the possessors of them. So that with much ado I was corrupted, and made to learn the dirty devices of this world." (72).[1]

This is a description of the attitude which Professor Piaget has named *egocentric*, seen from the inside. Piaget has shown

[1] Wordsworth's *Ode on Intimations of Immortality from Recollections of Early Childhood* may be compared with this but cannot have been directly influenced by it, since Traherne's work was not published till the present century.

how it does not seem strange to the egocentric child that the sun and moon should follow him when he goes out for a walk. This belief is not necessarily linked with a lack of some conception of death, for it was found to occur spontaneously, exactly as Piaget describes it, in one of the subjects of this research (Richard Clement when aged 5 : 8) at a time when he already had a conception of death. But in the child's early development the two are often co-existent. Traherne's recollections present the psychological matrix in which they co-exist. He shows egocentric ignorance as a positive and all-pervasive mental content, rather than as the negative thing or lacuna which ignorance commonly seems to the adult.

As there was no compulsion, so there was no death. As there was no death, so time was unknown. " And something infinite behind everything appeared," *which moved desire.* Here is perhaps the converse of many forms of mental disorder linked with the *failing* of desire " because man goeth to his long home " (5.*c*)—because things are found to be not infinite.

Notes on I

1. In these examples we may observe the concept of death as either non-existent or embryonic in the child's mind. They correspond roughly to Category A of the previous chapter. They lead us to consider more fully what mental experience or attitude provides the soil for the growth of the idea.

It appears very doubtful whether it can be derived from any uniform type of experience, objectively viewed. One child, puzzled by dead rabbits, thinks they are asleep ; another child actually thinks so of her dead mother yet she does not puzzle at all. One child is puzzled by the word " dead," another is attracted by a dramatic attitude associated with the word, but does not enquire further as to its meaning. One child is puzzled by a dead insect's cessation of movement and compares it with another animal's similar stillness.

The common factor here, in those whose experience is leading them to an embryonic conception of death, appears to be the attitude of puzzlement ; a reaction of wonder or surprise aroused by perception of dead things, or the use of the word. An anomaly or a gap has become apparent in the organization of their experience. Marlene's experience is not so organized as to lead her to demand a cause, or to be puzzled, when her mother suddenly falls down on the floor and seems asleep ; she is able to accept this as sleep or its equivalent. Stephen, on the other hand, is conscious of some anomaly when he perceives rabbits or poultry asleep and yet not asleep in shops. This stands out from the pattern of his experience as anomalous. Ben is at the stage of enquiring the meaning of the verbal symbol, as well as of the significance of the event in a very rudimentary way. Ursula is not puzzled by the verbal symbol, but by the features of the phenomenon itself, like Stephen.

The concept of death, then, does not begin to develop in the child's mind until there is already present (1) organization of experience at a certain level, and (2) some apprehension of causation. Roughly, he must have reached the *Why* stage.[1]

---

[1] Lewis (44) has pointed out that the use of *why* or *because* by the child does not always indicate appreciation of causal sequence, but that such appreciation may originate largely in the type of answer given by the adult to questions couched in this form. He is referring, however, to the earliest *why* questions, asked at under three years of age ; when the spate of *why's* begins, it indicates that the child *has* reached a stage when causal sequence is appreciated conceptually.

The degree of appreciation of causality indicated by the very earliest of a child's *why* questions may vary widely, however, and with some children the earliest *why's*, even if they refer to human behaviour, may refer clearly to an appreciation of anomaly demanding explanation. In this connection nothing could be more apt than the first *why* of Scupin's boy (quoted by Piaget and by N. Isaacs) : the child's mother was lying on the ground ; he wanted her to get up, and said, " Du bis ya nicht tot ; warum stehste nicht immersu auf ? "

To reach the *Why* stage : what does this imply ? At what stage of mental development does the child reach it, and what conditions his reaching it ? The question involves the problem of how the apprehension of cause arises : a problem not easy to solve, in spite of the amount of attention devoted to it.

Hume's famous, simple theory was that *post hoc* becomes *propter hoc* through association and habit. Things happen together constantly (the " togetherness," in space or time, being given, according to this and kindred theories, by attributes of the object independent of the experiencer) ; then they are expected to happen together ; and this is to look upon them as cause and effect. There is no real necessary relation between the phenomena, but only one of expectation, resulting from customary experience. Indeed, Hume argued, the principle of causation must be simple, since " the most ignorant and stupid peasants, nay infants, nay even brute beasts, act upon it " (31).

In modern terms we may say that Hume holds the idea of cause to be but a rationalization of conditioned reflex systems. Just as the brute beast's mouth will water at the sound of the bell which he is accustomed to hear shortly before his dinner comes, so man rationalizes similar " foresight " and calls his equivalent-of-the-bell the *cause* of his equivalent-of-the-dinner, according to Hume.

And indeed the experimenter on conditioned reflexes may refer to the sound of the bell as the cause of salivation in the beast ; but the animal can scarcely be said to apprehend a causal relationship between the two, although he may " act upon it." When the physiological functioning of infants is similarly " conditioned " to abnormal stimuli in the laboratory, the success of the experiments appears to depend on the child *not* seeking for any reason or causal relationship in his experience.

Stern has criticized Hume's theory of cause on the basis of observation of children's reactions in the normal course of development (64.i). He maintains that it is not expectation based on habitual experience that appears to give rise to the idea of cause in children, but the reversal of expectation. The concept of cause does not actually appear to originate (in Stern's observation) without a reaction expressive of wonder or surprise.

Does the child's conception of cause arise, then, from his discovery that he had, so to speak, acted on Hume's principle all along, and it was not sound ? Does he begin to conceive of cause when, having experienced phenomena in association many times, he finds them disappointingly dissociated—finds, for instance, " that one may smile, and smile, and be a villain ? "

Stern points out that even such a reversal of Hume's theory does not provide a satisfactory or sufficient explanation of children's behaviour, for they will seek to find causes for events and phenomena which are new in their experience; phenomena which they have not previously perceived in customary associations. Stern offers no solution of the problem this behaviour raises, but he quotes Helmholtz's suggestion that it arises from the child's *unconscious conclusions.*

Analyzed in the terms Spearman would use, such an unconscious conclusion would derive from an apprehension of causal relationship existing unconsciously, between a consciously-perceived datum of experience (the effect) and an unknown, unexperienced correlate (sought as cause). Spearman has pointed out that there may be apprehension of causal relationship even when the data perceived as cause or effect have not actually or have only partially this relation to each other in reality (61.i).

But to trace an apprehension of causal relationship into the unconscious mind is not to discover its genesis in individual development. For that, material must be sought in the behaviour of the very young infant, and the responsive-interpretative behaviour of its mother.[1] The new-born baby's cry is a kind of pointless yowling, testifying to his condition rather than his desires. As the days go on, the mother notices a different kind of sound, expressing to her ears anger or impatience ; then, after a few weeks, other tones still are distinguished, which she interprets as constituting a demand, made with intention. The grizzling unhappiness of the earliest days is now superseded. It is clear that the infant apprehends himself as a power, an agent. The mother may even profess to find herself ruled by a tyrant with all the manners of a dictator. Of the existence of the intention and the effort to bring things about, the baby's behaviour leaves no doubt whatever now in the mother's mind. Here is an early foundation for the apprehension of causation.

M. Piaget attributes to Maine de Biran the earliest statement of the theory that consciousness of inner force, entering experience through sensations of muscular innervation, originates the idea of force in general, or cause. Piaget himself believes that the apprehension of causality has a dual source, and derives from experience both of the self as a force, and of external objects as forces, each of these (the self and the external things) being interpreted in terms of the other. He thus holds a balance even between the derivation of the causal idea from projection and introjection, and draws an illuminating parallel between these complementary mental activities and the adaptive and assimilative processes by which the life of biological organisms is physiologically maintained.

Biran's suggestion that the idea of cause derives from the sense of self's force is incorporated by Piaget into his own fuller theory, but Piaget first subjects it to criticism, on both

[1] I believe that the behaviour of the infant and a mother who nurses and constantly cares for it may be considered as a psychological unit for purposes of interpretation. What the infant's behaviour means to the mother is believed to correlate closely with what it means to him.

empirical and theoretical grounds, which seems less justified than his final (qualified) adoption of it. Thus he writes :

" According to Maine de Biran . . . force is first of all grasped in the self and then inferred in external objects. . . . Now, if we confront this process thought out by Maine de Biran with the facts . . . we are led to an exact reversal of the order of things. For everything happens as though the child began by attributing forces to all outside bodies, and as though he only ended by finding himself the ' I ' that was the cause of his own force.

" After all, nothing is less likely than that the feeling of self should originate in very young children. . . . All that we have seen (*i.e.*, during M. Piaget's researches) . . . seems rather to indicate that our earliest experiences are not referred to a central ' I,' but float about in an undifferentiated absolute. The self would thus be the result of a gradual and progressive dissociation, and not of a primitive intuition "(53.*b*.i).

Objections may be raised to each of these arguments. To the first : that M. Piaget's " facts " are derived from the responses of children already too old for their behaviour to refute or establish a theory about the earliest modes of apprehension of cause by Biran's theory. Indeed M. Piaget has himself said that his theories about the causal apprehensions of younger infants are deductions from his observations on older children (aged 3 to 11 years), not inductions from directly observed fact (53.*b*.ii). " We can learn enough from the laws of evolution (of the conception of causality) between 3 and 11 years," he writes, " and there is no need to attach any special importance to the original stage."

But instead of extending M. Piaget's deductions on the older child to cover the infant, we may attempt to discover whether observation of the infant himself does actually confirm the general direction of evolution which M. Piaget indicates. For it has been argued, with evidence from other observations, for instance by Dr. Susan Isaacs (44.*a*), that

Piaget's conclusions about the older child's notions of causality are themselves not to be accepted without question.

Observations of other child-psychologists suggest that the young child does, in a certain special sense, very definitely refer his experiences to an " I " which is by no means an undifferentiated absolute. The apprehension of self-as-agent appears to arise during the first year of life, before speech. Many observers have recorded how the baby behaves as though he were enjoying being a doer, when, for instance, he repeatedly bangs a spoon on a table ; he gives the impression that his motive is to make things happen, and to be conscious of himself-as-doing-it.

Psychology in Biran's day would find it necessary to derive the consciousness of self-as-agent from the consciousness of self as a distinct functional entity. Mental processes were conceived as being built up from elements that were characterized by a simpler structure *in the thought of the psychologist*. We do not now suppose that that which seems simpler or elementary in our thinking is necessarily prior in development. The psychologist of to-day does not therefore need to reject Biran's suggestion that the apprehension of cause arises from the sense of self's effort, on the ground that the self is not dissociated or become conscious at such an early age. In the light of recent studies of the mode of growth of whole and parts of organisms, the consciousness of self-as-agent may now be accepted as a development prior to the full consciousness of self as such, and the apprehension of cause may be judged to derive largely (though not entirely, for its origin may be dual, as M. Piaget holds) from the consciousness of self-as-agent, originating with the cries of the baby in the cradle.

The discovery of agency, however, whether it is first apprehended as inherent in external or internal " forces " (either of which must be preceded by *some* apprehension of the self) brings the child no higher than the animal or perceptual level. He has still far to go before he reaches a

WHY stage. In that progress, three different processes may be seen at work, bringing him on his way to the conception of cause.

First, is *the increasing range and complexity of the organization of experience*. The perception of cause arises within a scheme which includes an *end* and a *means* : as for instance, the *end* of being fed, and the *means* of making a noise. In order to fix such a perception stably in the mind as a relationship, and give it general application, it is necessary that ends should be various. The widening of the range of ends, or interests, is the spontaneous accompaniment of general mental maturation. Thus the development of the concept of cause depends on the whole of mental development. As the baby's interest progresses towards a more various range of objects—lights and faces, voices, rattles, the movements of his own body and the sound of his own voice—so the percept of causal relationship develops towards a concept. *Cause* becomes any actively helping or hindering medium to a desired end. It ceases to be bound up in crying and food. It begins to be generalized.

Second, is *the development of surprise*. The perception of cause only arises where there is organization of interest. Outside the range of interest there can be no surprise at any occurrence. Surprise is founded on the reversal of expectation, conscious or unconscious. Unconscious expectation is explicable if we suppose it to be founded on identification of objects within the interest scheme : if X brings about Y (or appears in a *Gestalt* with Y), then this experience X′ (identified in the unconscious with X) will bring about Y′ (likewise identified with Y). The identification only occurs when the subject has been sufficiently interested in X′ to substitute it mentally for X. The process may be conceived as a displacement of affect due to X on to the new X′ ; the affect is identical, and so its objects are identified—just as to hunger, all appropriate objects are alike *food*. The displacement of affect is made on the understanding that X′ will

behave in material respects as X did.[1] The interest in X'
thus includes interest in seeing whether X' does behave as
X did—that is, whether Y' does appear, too. Interest is
thus led to the *functional difference* between X and X'. Cause
is not only generalized but also *abstracted* from the physical
objects in which it is made manifest, and is apprehended as
something intangible.

Hence also arises a questioning and analysis of causative
properties of things which, as Stout (65) points out, marks
the difference between perceptual and ideational apprehension of cause, and also the difference between the more
primitive and the more civilized attitude.

Outside the child's field of interest—that is, the range of
objects covered by such affect-displacements—the most
unusual things may happen without his paying them the
slightest attention. They will not serve to develop his idea
of cause. Within his range of interest, expectation (conscious
or unconscious) will serve in this way. Either confirmation
or reversal of expectation will strengthen the apprehension
of cause ; reversal particularly will turn him back to a
further seeking for means, a further analysis of properties of
things, a further exploration of whole situations.

Third comes a process which develops comparatively late.
It consists in a re-enactment on the ideational plane of
behaviour previously acted out at the perceptual level ; that
is, the abandonment of the practice of simply vocalizing
wants as a means to their fulfilment, and the substitution of
the attempt to organize other means to secure satisfaction,
such as, for instance, one's own other motor powers, and the
properties of objects which these other powers may make
available. This is the process which, *in its later re-enactment*,
ushers in the *Why* stage.

---

[1] An over-simplification has been made here. The displacement may
be due to ambivalence towards X' so that X' is identified with one
aspect of X only (*e.g.*, good-X) and expected Y is good-Y, not Y wholly
identified.

I

That the *Why* stage is one due to spontaneous maturation
rather than to accidents of experience is obvious to those who
have the opportunity to observe the phenomenon in several
children. The stage of *Why* questioning follows after a stage
of *What* questioning, sometimes through an intervening
stage of *What for* (*e.g.*, What for did Daddie buy a new hat ?)
The child may have the opportunity of hearing *Why*
questions and causal reasoning used by others around him ;
and he is capable of pronouncing the word *Why* as early as
What ; but he does not develop the *Why* attitude to
experience in general so early as the *What* attitude. He has
used causation in his actions ; he has nibbled at the idea in
speech ; but until the full *Why* stage dawns, he has yet to
apprehend it in that fullness which results in the intoxication
with the idea of causation characteristic of the elder-toddler
stage, beginning at about the beginning of the fourth year
of life.

During the previous *What* or *Who* stage, the child is deeply
occupied with learning word symbols which may give more
exact vocal definition to his desires. He has grasped the
essential idea of verbal symbolism and conventional
significance—an idea which came to the blind girl, Helen
Keller, late enough for her to introspect and record the
surprised delight which marks an intellectual crisis, a new
insight. The applications of that insight occupy the child,
and there for a time he pauses. So far as the conception of
cause is concerned he is still using words in the way he used
cries in the cradle, when his grizzling had changed to an
angry, intended demand. He has gained in the dis-
criminatory fineness of this same vocal power ; names help ;
he can call precisely whom he wants, ask for what he wants,
even, later, explain what is wrong in a situation. But after
a while he begins to discover the limitations of this new
power. People do not only withhold what he wants because
they do not understand that he wants it. The old plan to
get what he wants by crying out for it, and the new plan to

get it more surely and precisely by learning the names of people and things, have both a flaw. People may learn what he wants, and not do it. The power it gives him is only indirect and contingent.[1]

Now, the child from a very early age has achieved some of his desires not by calling for help, but by direct intelligent action. He begins, before he can speak, to link cognitive data in such a way that he is able to get what he wants, recognizing and circumventing obstruction. He realizes himself as an effective agent through other effectors than the vocal muscles. There comes a stage when language has been mastered, and yet found not to be a talisman, when this new instrument, word-thought, is applied in the more advanced way, as a mental tool for self-help. This is when causality begins to be apprehended as an ideal relation between phenomena. This apprehension of cause arises from a conceptual evaluation of means, parallel to the perceptual evaluation by which the baby in Karl Bühler's experiment managed to secure the rusk, and the apes in Köhler's experiments secured their bananas. The child has now come to the stage when he seeks to effect desires, or to make a satisfactory organization of experience prospectively, through understanding the causal relations of phenomena conceptually. By generalization of the causal idea, from the variety of things perceived to behave alike in so far as they are agents or means, and by abstraction of it, through apprehension of functional differences between things which might otherwise be substituted for each other, the relation-

---

[1] In attributing to the child the attitude of expecting to get what he wants just by knowing how to use words to ask for it, we are crediting him with that " autism " which M. Piaget has described. The child is showing a blindness to the existence of a world with a will different from his own. The suggestion here made, however, is somewhat different from M. Piaget's. It is suggested that the new power of language leads the child for a time to take up this attitude again as his prevailing one, but that never after his earliest infancy does it hold the mental field alone.

ship itself becomes a separable mental object, to which separable word-sounds apply. " Why " and " because " are the commonest of these words. Their use by others, heard by the child, encourages the maturing of the causal idea, but his own intoxication with them comes as a definite stage in his mental progress. It marks his passing from that stage (to which he and we may frequently regress) of attempting to gain his ends through the power inherent in words, to a state when he attempts to gain all by understanding and influencing and using potencies and motives and reasons— functional differences in things and people. In both stages he seems to have an immensely exaggerated view of the power (or, if he is an anxious child, the security) which would be his if he could completely control these weapons— words, in the earlier stage, causal understanding (largely through words) in the latter.

It seems that the attachment of meaning to the word " dead," or the definite idea of death as a distinctive thing, does not arise before this stage of development. Observation suggests that this is so, but does not provide an explanation of it. Only a theoretical explanation can be offered. It is that the What stage is concerned with things, simply, whereas the Why stage is concerned with the functioning of things. No simple " thing " meaning can be attached to *dead* or death ; it can only have meaning as function. Dead and death cannot present themselves to the child as things, nor even as conditions of things, except negatively. There- fore apprehension of their meaning must be preceded not only by the long mental development that leads to the appreciation of verbal symbolism, but also by the application of verbal symbols to functions and functional differences ; that is, it can only come at the Why stage.

2. Ben's inability to understand what was meant by the word *dead* is interesting in the light of an earlier record of the same boy when he was ten months younger (2 : 4).

This showed that his criteria for distinguishing living and not-living objects were very hazy.

(The mother's record) : I took Ben to tea at his grandmother's house, and she got a large doll out of a drawer. Ben seemed to think it was alive ; he took it in his arms, put his face to its face, and then said, " Mummie kiss it." He wanted me to kiss it, but he himself always calls me " mother." When I undressed it for him, he still thought it real, and excitedly showed it pictures. When we came home, we got out a smaller doll, which would not open and shut its eyes, and then after a time he realized it was a toy, and I think realized at the same time about the other doll. He never showed much interest in dolls after that.

II.—*The child's earliest concept of death may be very limited, or erroneous.*

EXAMPLES. (*a*) *Home Records.*

(i) *Richard, aged 3 : 11*
(An independent summary of political affairs on the occasion of the accession of Edward VIII. Richard was sitting on his mother's lap being dried after his bath :)
" The old king is dead, and he's married ; the new king is not dead, and he's not married."

(ii) *Francis, aged 4 : 5*
Francis was examining a pictorial Bible while he was alone with me (M.) in the drawing-room of his grandparents' house one day. He was particularly interested in a picture of the death of Moses, which represented Moses kneeling on a mountain with a bright light directed on to him. Francis asked what the picture was about, and I read the title. He exclaimed in surprise, " Is that how you die ? " I explained that we all did not die like that. He remained puzzled, and afterwards the picture seemed to have a great fascination for him, for he turned to it whenever he had the opportunity.

(iii) *Francis, aged 4 : 10*
Francis was having lunch alone with his mother, and said

in a conversation about the king, " Do kings always die with their crowns on ? "   He was told " No," and then said, " How do you know when people are going to die ? " and was told, " They generally become very weak and ill."   He then changed the subject.

(iv) *Stephen, aged 4 : 10 (further from his mother's letter, already quoted, p. 102).*

At present he thinks that we all turn into statues when we die, owing to the fact that he first met Queen Victoria as a statue in Kensington Gardens and then was told that she had been dead some time.

(v) *Stephen, aged 4 : 11*

Stephen was getting into pyjamas before the nursery fire alone with M., and looking at a picture of a fountain—a statue of a girl pouring water.

S. : Mummie, what's that lady doing ?

M. : That's not really a lady, it's a statue.

S. : Perhaps she's just died.

M. explained that he made a mistake when he was a little boy about Queen Victoria's statue.   People make statues out of stone to look like people ; they're not real people at all and never have been.   S. changed the subject completely but showed no emotion at all—to all appearances just forgot about it.

EXAMPLES.   (*b*) *From published literature.*

(i) *Julius Katz, aged 3 : 10 ; Theodor, aged 5 : 5* (35.ii)

J. : If people don't go out for a walk, they die.

T. : People don't die if they don't go out for a walk, but they grow pale.

(ii) *Ruth Rasmussen, aged 4 plus* (55.*a*.ii)

Ruth's grandfather, of whom she was very fond, died when she was four.   This made, however, no immediate impression on her.   She asked why she should not go to the funeral.   " Why not ? Does grandpa mind ? "

Notes on II

The characteristic feature of this group is that the concept is limited, rather than that it is erroneous or uncertain. Error will be found under other headings as well, but when it is combined with elaboration of the concept it would not be included in this group.

The group as a whole corresponds with Category B of the definitions.

It is noted by the mothers on several occasions that the child, after raising the subject of death, or having it referred to, himself then changed the subject ; sometimes it is added, as with Stephen above, that he showed no emotion. Such reports suggest a certain quality of interest in the subject on the child's part. There may be repression of emotion ; or there may be a wish to defer the receiving of more information until the information just received has been welded into the existent organization of knowledge. Such doubtful points are only to be decided by observation of the child's behaviour over a long period of time. The mother's statement that the child showed no emotion is not to be taken as proof that the child felt none. An emotional reaction (at this same age), which seems a very " normal " one, is reported by Rasmussen of his daughter, Sonia :

Sonia Rasmussen, aged 4 : 7 (55.b.i)
S. had heard that a little girl was dead, and said, " How sad it is for that little girl that she is dead. I would be very sorry, too, if it was me that was dead."

III.—*Bodily actions associated with the concept of death.*

Children may act on ideas of death, or perform actions which influence their ideas, before they express such ideas clearly in words. A very great number of games handed down in the culture of the nursery contain activities of this kind. Apart from these, we found children displaying individual differences in bodily behaviour connected with the idea, which were remarkably consistent, and roughly resolved themselves into two antithetical types, distinguished as follows :—

A type : Avoidance of contact with dead things, or of any
　　　　responsibility for the event.
B type : Enjoyment of killing.

Type A children at a later stage tend to object to the
killing of animals for sport, and sometimes also for food ;
they may become vegetarian.　Type B children (so far as
they were observed during this research) do not seem to
think of giving pain, or find their enjoyment in that ; they
appear to seek reassurances of their own power, offensive and
defensive.

The home records show distinctive A characteristics in
three children, Catherine, Ben and Judith, and B
characteristics in two, Richard and Timothy.　Two young
friends of these children, David and Jean, also seemed to
possess B characteristics.　It was noted, though it may be
mere coincidence, that all the A children were elder siblings,
and all the B children but Jean (who was an only child)
were younger ones.　Sully's record of his boy Clifford,
however, shows him as distinctly A type, but he was a
second child.

The present group of examples aim at illustrating these
contrasted types of motor behaviour associated with the
concept of death, and also the consistency of attitude shown
by individual children.　More space has been given to the
aggressive type (B), because it is socially disapproved and
consequently is less adequately recorded in previous studies.

EXAMPLES.　(*a*) *From Home Records.*

(i) *Judith, 7 : 6, and Timothy, 3 : 11*
After rain Judith and Timothy found a washed-up worm.
Judith said, " Don't tread on it, Timothy ; it may not be
dead." Timothy said, " I like it to be dead," and trod on it.
(This is the only relevant record for these siblings.)

(ii) *Ben, aged 3 : 3*
Ben picked some buttercups and then immediately threw
them away.　M. suggested it was a pity not to keep them,

but he said no, he wouldn't keep them, " 'cos they'll go dead."[1]

(iii) *Catherine, aged 6 : 9 (this entry, made when the record was opened, referred to an earlier occurrence).*

I (M.) was reading to Catherine one evening, after she was in bed at about 6.30, as was my custom. The book in question was *Nellie's Teachers*, a rather old-fashioned children's story. A visit to a death-bed by two little girls was being described. Catherine was listening with interest and attention, but quite cheerfully, until she heard that the little girls bent in turn to kiss the brow of the dead woman. She at once exclaimed in horror and disgust that anyone should wish to kiss a dead body, the idea of corruption appearing to be uppermost in her mind. She seemed to have no sense of horror at death itself, appearing to regard it as natural and inevitable, but she regarded it as " disgusting " (this was the word used) that anyone should touch a dead body in this intimate way.

(iv) *Catherine Holland, aged 9 : 2 ; Susanna Holland, aged 7 : 0 ; and Richard Clement, aged 5 : 11*

Catherine and Susanna were playing " sardines " out of doors with Richard and his mother. After one seeking, when we had all found each other, we stayed idly sitting under a hedge. C., poking about in the dry leaves with a stick, found a little bundle that looked like a bit of a bird's nest ; she said it was a dead bird, and then by looking closely M. saw that it was : there were a few wing bones sticking out at one side, and a dried claw.

C. went on to say how she found a tiny dead bird in the garden recently, and buried it in a match-box : it was very tiny and yellow (probably embryonic), but you could see it was a bird because of the bones, " like the ones you see in

---

[1] This entry was made less than two months after that already quoted on p. 102. To the present entry the following observation was added : Ben has been for about three months at the *Why* stage, very continuous and persistent. One day he said, " Why do I say why, mother ? " Another entry records his asking, at the end of a string of *why* questions, " Why all things ? "

museums." " And then I dug it up," she said several times, apparently meaning that she exhumed the buried bird.

Susanna made to touch the dead bird before us on the ground, but Catherine quickly said, " No, don't touch it ; it might have been dead a long time, and then it's not nice to touch." She poked at it again with her stick. Richard observed and listened, but said nothing.

(v) *Richard Clement, a series of entries in chronological order :*
Aged 3 : 0

An entry states : Richard drowned the kitten in the water-glass bin. The statement is then amplified : more correctly, R. threw the kitten into the bin, which had had preserved eggs in it and at the time contained only some thick liquid at the bottom. He then threw in a teddy-bear. Then he ran round the house whimpering and calling for someone to come and help to get them out. By the time M. came to the rescue the kitten was dead. M. was very much distressed. She despatched Richard to the nursery in the care of a maid before beginning to fish the bodies out of the chemical. As R. was led upstairs he asked for his bear and burst into tears when told he could not have it yet. (Actually the bear, though hung out to dry, was no use any more.)

M. was anxious that Richard should not be made to feel guilt or fear through his elder brother's reactions to this event, and she was able to get another kitten from the same litter without Ben knowing of what had happened. Richard did not tell Ben, though he knew the difference between the two kittens himself. The second kitten did not settle down, although kindly treated.

Previous entries about Richard and the first kitten show that he was nervous of it, though it was very small indeed. " R. runs round it, saying, ' He won't hurt me, he won't hurt me,' and keeping his toes carefully out of the kitten's reach."

Aged 4 : 7

R. : I killed the black cat. I cut it in half in the coal shed, with a chopper.

M. : Oh, why did you do that ?

R. : I thought we didn't want it any more.

M. : Could I see the body ?

R. : No, it isn't there now. I stucked it together again, and it walked away.

(M.'s note : We have no cat, but I believe there was a cat which called on us casually at this time, and R. was interested in it.)

Aged 5 : 1

There was a drowsy bee crawling about us when we were having tea in the garden, and M. brushed it off Richard ; we all watched it with interest for quite a long time. Finally R. said he would tread on it.

M. : Don't ; it won't hurt you if you leave it alone.

But a little later, when nobody was paying much attention to him, R. did tread on it, and seemed pleased with himself.

Aged 5 : 3

M., out for a walk with R., heard rather indistinctly a sentence : " Jean and I . . . go out for a walk . . . find ants, to tread on them." (Jean is a friend of R.'s, a year younger.)

Aged 5 : 4

Cutting open a cooking-apple, M. found an earwig in it. R. wanted her to kill it, but she did not want to. He was very keen to kill it himself. M. caught it in a piece of paper and gave it to him. He took it out on the kitchen step, and a knife, and squashed or cut it. (M. did not watch this.) He then returned cheerfully to the kitchen, saying : " It moved, very slowly, the first time after it was dead ; why did it do that, Mother ? " He then returned and cut it into little bits, and came back into the kitchen with the knife.

Ben Clement, aged 8 : 6, Richard Clement, aged 5 : 4, and David, a friend, also 5 : 4.

All having tea together ; Mrs. C. also present.

David : I love wasps. Because we kill them. (He has a beaming smile as he speaks. The wasps fly around.)

Ben : Oh, do you ? I don't. One stung me once, on the nose.

Richard (beaming like David) : Yes, I love killing things, too.

Ben : I hate killing things. . . . (He went on with a long announcement of non-aggressive sentiments, with a reference to Nature, which could not be recorded owing to the necessity for administering food.)

Ben, aged 9 : 1, and Richard, aged 5 : 11. (In the garden with F. ; overheard and recorded by M.)

R. : Here's a nice thin worm.

B. (angrily) : Why did you kill him ? . . . You mustn't do that ; it hurts them, doesn't it ? (to F.).

F. : Yes. . . .

R. : It doesn't matter with *worms.* . . . I like to watch them.

F. : Well, then, *watch* them.

B. : That one's gone suddenly long.

Richard, aged 6 : 1

M. and Richard found a wood-louse in the earth while gardening. R. was delighted, and carried it off to the porch step on a trowel. He watched it for about a quarter of an hour, hedging it off from escaping, and then said he wanted to keep it in a box. M. said that would be rather cruel to it ; it would not like to be away from the ground. This did not deter R., who went up to the nursery and got a tin with a lid. He put the insect in this and then was fetched to bed. As he went upstairs he was heard to say, " I do like being cruel to animals."

In these children's spontaneous behaviour we find expressed two essential motives of primitive religion : the untouchableness of the dead, which may be an origin of sacredness, taboo, and is undoubtedly connected with it ; and the ambivalence towards the victim of aggression—the assertion of love for the victim—which is a marked feature of many totem rites.

The instance of Ben deciding to throw away the flowers he had only just picked shows that the avoidance of contact with the dead may be quite independent of any immediate unpleasant sensory quality in the object. With David there could be no doubt of the correct use of " because," when he said he loved wasps " because we kill them." Richard cordially supported David when he expressed this sentiment, and the faces of both these charming little boys beamed and dimpled with pleasure.

Richard was never heard to express affection for animals used for food, on the ground that we eat them. The love for wasps, worms, etc., obviously arose from the gratification they gave to the desire for consciousness of power.[1]

The question of the importance of animals in the development of the child's concept of death will be considered more fully later.

Catherine's behaviour on hearing of the children kissing the dead woman might suggest that the corpse was equated with fæces, as psycho-analysts say that it often is in the unconscious mind. The behaviour of Judith and Ben did not suggest this equation. Freud (21.*b*.ii) has noted associations between fæces (looked on with favour as an external object produced by the self)—considered as potential gifts—hence equated with money, or with *flowers*, or with children. Here we have Catherine " disgusted " at anyone coming into intimate contact with the dead, and Ben averse to contact with flowers because they will die. We have, however, no evidence of what is primary in the associations which lead to these reactions, in the case of Catherine and Ben.

EXAMPLES. (*b*) *From published literature.*

Sully gives an example of motor behaviour at a very early age, relative to the development of the concept of death,

---

[1] Richard, it is recorded, enjoyed chasing chickens, and even geese, but did not then express affection for them. He became very fond of a dog at one time (aged 6 : 4), and afterwards wrote it letters. He was never known to bully other children.

which may conflict with the above hypothesis of complete differentiation of types ; alternatively, it may be an instance of behaviour previous to differentiation. The home records have no instance of this kind of behaviour combined with verbal expression at such an early age :

"A little boy (aged 2 : 2), after nearly killing a fly on the window-pane, seemed surprised and disturbed, looking round for an explanation, then gave it himself : ' Mr. F'y dom (gone) to by-by.' But he would not touch it or another fly again—a doubt evidently remained and he continued uneasy about it. Here we have the instinctive attitude of a child towards the outcome of his destructive impulse. This impulse is not necessarily cruel in the sense of including an idea of the animal's suffering " (66.i).

Sully's account of his own boy's reactions to the idea of death shows the boy (Clifford) as a consistent A type. Since the A type seek to avoid contact with and responsibility for death, their motor behaviour does not so easily provide examples of their attitude, and most of Sully's relevant references are to verbal rather than motor behaviour. A few may be selected :

" C., *when only four*, was moved to passionate grief at the sight of a dead dog taken from a pond."
Aged 3 : 6
He was at this time, like other children, much troubled about the killing of animals for food. Again and again he would ask with something of fierce impatience in his voice : " *Why* do people kill them? " . . . He contended that people who eat meat must like animals to be killed. Finally, to clinch the matter, he turned on his mother and asked, " Do *you* like them to be killed ? "
Aged 4 : 4
(Looking at a picture book of animals, *à propos* of a picture of seals :)

C. : What are seals killed for, Mamma ?

M. : For the sake of their skins and oil.

C. (turning to a picture of a stag) : Why do they kill the stags ? They don't want their skins, do they ?

M. : No, they kill them because they like to chase them.

C. : Why don't policemen stop them ?

M. : They can't do that, because people are allowed to kill them.

C. (loudly and passionately) : Allowed, allowed ? People are not allowed to take other people and kill them.

M. : People think there is a difference between killing men and killing animals.

C. was not to be pacified this way. He looked woebegone, and said to his mother piteously, " You don't understand me."

An entry on the following page records that he broke off his toy soldiers' guns " when I thought they were just naughty men who liked to kill people " (66.ii).

Shakespeare describes, in *Coriolanus*, behaviour of B type in Coriolanus' little son. The description gives an indication of intentional cruelty which is undoubtedly to be observed at times in children's actions to animals. In these records we have come nearest to it in Richard's treatment of the wood-louse, earwig and worms ; the impression then given, in spite of Richard's own testimony, was that he did not consider the animal as suffering pain at all.

Valeria : How does your little son ?

Virgilia (Coriolanus' wife) : I thank your ladyship ; well, good madam.

Volumnia (Coriolanus' mother) : He had rather see the swords, and hear a drum, than look upon his schoolmaster.

Valeria : O' my word, the father's son ; I'll swear, 'tis a very pretty boy. O' my troth, I looked upon him o' Wednesday half an hour together : he has such a confirmed countenance. I saw him run after a gilded butterfly ; and when he caught it, he let it go again ; and after it again ;

and over and over he comes, and up again ; catched it
again : or whether his fall enraged him, or how 'twas, he
did so set his teeth, and tear it : O, I warrant, how he
mammocked it !

Volumnia : One of his father's moods. (60.*d*).

It is not difficult to understand why we have few references
to this sort of behaviour in books on Child Psychology, for
the observer can seldom remain merely observant of it.
Mrs. Isaacs gives a number of instances of children's cruelty
to animals by which we are also enabled to see the strong
resultant reaction of the social environment upon the child
(33.*a*.iii).

11.5.25. Harold found another dead rat in the garden.
He and Frank stamped on it. (*Harold,* 5 : 3 ; Frank,
5 : 6.)

22.5.25. When the children were changing the water of
the gold-fish, Frank had a sudden impulse of cruelty and
said to the others, " Shall we stamp on it ? " Mrs. I. did
not imagine that they would really do this, and when they
ran out into the garden with it, she followed after them, but
not quite quickly enough. Before she could stop them they
had thrown the fish out into the sand and stamped on it.
They stood round and looked at it, rather excited, and
obviously wishing they hadn't done it, and Frank said,
" Now let's put it into water, and then it'll come alive
again." They put it back into the water, but soon saw that
it was dead, and later on they buried it in the sand. All
the children, including the instigator, Frank, were obviously
full of regret at having done this, and a wish that they had
the fish back again. (N.B.—This was the only incident of
its kind in the school.)

The impulse to stamp or tread on a dead animal, or to
kill it in this way, was also shown by Timothy (see p. 120),
Richard, as already recorded on p. 123 (aged 5 : 1), and
again by *Richard, aged 5 : 3 :*

M. found a dead mouse in the garden, and told R. He was much interested.

M. : Don't touch it, except with a stick.

R. : Can I tread on it ? Can it feel ? Can it see ?

He prodded it, asking questions the while. M. turned it over with the stick. He showed no repulsion, nor pity (M. suggested none, by voice or manner).[1] His behaviour gave an impression of genuine interest, mixed with disappointment that a small animal which was at his mercy, unable to run away, yet could not be an object for a display of power on his part. There was no impression given that he wished to cause it *pain*.

Richard's account of how he and Jean sought for ants, to tread on them, occurred later in the same day (see p. 120).

Notes to III

In suggesting that there are two antithetical types of motor behaviour relative to the death concept, it is not implied that all instances of aggressiveness can be brought under the same head. Children may behave aggressively in such a way as to cause the death of animals, when the death is actually an incidental result. Their behaviour is not then primarily motivated by or connected with their attitude to death, and may consequently run quite contrary to their type as orientated by their death concept and attitude. Hence although A type will seldom behave cruelly, and B type may often (from the objective point of view) do so (and may grow to find cruelty itself a pleasure in later years), their behaviour in this respect may be inconsistent. When it is inconsistent, the ruling motive will probably be clearly

---

[1] The mother, however, evidently suggested the untouchableness of the dead animal to the child, to whom it appears that the idea would not (in this case) have occurred spontaneously.

The same observer elsewhere records a boy as having run into the house from the garden holding in his hand a dead baby mole, to show to her and another boy, and how this boy commented on the first for having picked up the dead animal in his hand.

K

apparent. The proviso of inconsistency is made rather of instances given in literature ; not of the home records children, who (if we remember that cruelty is not the *aim* of the B's so that fondness for animals is not inconsistent) were remarkably consistent in their attitudes and behaviour in this respect.

Mrs. Isaacs, for example, gives an instance of behaviour apparently very cruel on the part of a little girl usually kind to animals. It is clear that the child on this occasion does not connect the cruel action with a concept of death, and is too much excited by other impulses to consider the animal as a sentient thing except in so far as that fact makes more repulsive the task she sets to her suitors :

Priscilla, aged 6 : 6
" The children went into the garden. Priscilla wanted to pull a worm into halves, and said she would marry the boy who did. They all said they wanted to marry her. Dan eventually did pull the worm in halves. Frank then pulled the rest of it apart ; they were very excited about this. (It should be noted how few instances of actual cruelty are recorded against Priscilla.) " (33.*b*.)

IV.—*Errors arise through misunderstanding of cultural teaching.*

EXAMPLES.   (*a*) *From Home Records.*

Francis, aged 4 : 11
Francis was out for a walk with M. and the baby. There was some conversation about holly which he had picked.
F. : Flowers die and we die, don't we, Mummy ?
M. : Yes.
F. : Who kills us in the night ? Does Jesus ?
M. : We die when we are old or ill, or if some sudden accident occurs.
F. : Like lepers, for lepers are diseased, aren't they ? They go white, with spots on their legs.
Note in the record : The reference to Jesus killing us in the night is due, I think, to the fact that Francis has recently

had read to him the nursery rhyme about " Matthew, Mark, Luke and John," in which the following lines occur :

> Before I lay me down to sleep
> I give my soul to Christ to keep,
> And if I die before I wake,
> I pray that Christ my soul will take.

No comment was made at the time.

It is often possible to observe a weaving together of the beliefs suggested by traditional teaching, and those growing out of the child's own directive thought, in which the cultural beliefs seem to provide a woof of fantasy. For instance :

Ben, aged 6 : 4

B. : Why can't you keep cream to the next day ?

M. : Because it goes bad. Most things do that have been alive ; if you don't eat them soon, you can't eat them at all.

B. : Do you think when we die we go up to the shops in Heaven, and then God buys us and puts us in his larder and eats us ?

Richard, aged 5 : 5 (1937)

As R. and M. walked up from the beach, R. talked at great length, beginning with rational discussion of coming bad weather, and going on with obvious fantasy : " lightning —thunder is drums of soldiers in the sky—we shall go up in the sky if a war comes, so you needn't mind—the angels will let down a long rope with a hook on the end, and catch you up on the hook (this was addressed to M. personally), and then you'll turn into an angel, and it will be lovely, 'cos you'll able to fly—because angels can fly, they have wings."

There was also a reference to God in the sky, and to there being some who doubt His existence, but the doubt was set aside as negligible.[1]

EXAMPLES. (b) *From published literature.*

Rasmussen speaks of the child's interest in death as resulting from their " hearing relevant subjects mentioned."

---

[1] Note by M. written down immediately on arrival at the house.

It is only in exceptional cases (he says) that one is content with letting the child know that the dead are buried or burnt ; as a rule one adds that the dead are with God in heaven, a statement that the child interprets in a grossly animistic manner. " Thus once when I was digging in my garden and by chance covered up a worm, a small boy who was watching me said, ' Now it will go up to Our Lord.' " (55.*a*.ii).

The Malting House School children had helped to bury a dead rabbit. The next day, two of the boys

" talked of digging the rabbit up," but *Frank* (5 : 9) said, " It's not there—it's gone up to the sky." They began to dig, but tired of it, and ran off to something else. Later they came back, and dug again. *Duncan* (7 : 2), however, said, " Don't bother—it's gone—it's up in the sky," and gave up digging. Mrs. I. therefore said, " Shall we see if it's there ? " and also dug. They found the rabbit, and were very interested to see it still there. (33.*a*.iv)

Such examples could, of course, be easily multiplied. They are particularly common in the form of jokes about childish sayings.

Notes on IV

The attitude of these children to traditional teaching about the after-life is very much like that Malinowski has described in primitive peoples :

" It is possible to put all these questions to the natives, the most intelligent of whom will grasp them without difficulty and discuss them with the ethnographer, showing a considerable amount of insight and interest. But such discussions have proved to me unmistakably that in dealing with these and similar questions one leaves behind the domain of belief proper and approaches quite a different class of native ideas. Here the native speculates rather than positively believes, and his speculations are not a very serious matter to him, nor does he trouble at all as to whether they are orthodox or not. Only exceptionally intelligent natives will enter into such questions at all, and these express rather their private opinion than positive tenets.

. . . When forced against a metaphysical wall by such questions as ' How can a *baloma*[1] call out, and eat, and make love if it is like a *saribu* (reflection) ' . . . the more intelligent replied (that the *baloma* were also like men). The less intelligent or less patient informants were inclined to shrug their shoulders over such questions ; others, again, would obviously become interested in the speculations, and produce extempore opinions, and ask your view, and just enter into a metaphysical discussion of a sort." (48.*a*.i)

Children likewise will often enjoy embroidering or speculating on the traditional beliefs about Heaven, or will enter into metaphysical discussion with pleasure. As for shrugging the shoulders, Sully has a pleasant example of the attitude :

C., aged 4 : 10
continued to ask how God made things, and wanted to know whether " preachers " could resolve his difficulty. . . . On learning . . . (that they might not be able to do so) he observed : " Well, anyhow, if we go to heaven when we die we shall know," and added, after a pause, " and if we don't, it doesn't much matter." (66.iii)

---

[1] A spirit of the dead.

CHAPTER VII

DEATH, BIRTH AND HOSTILITY

AFTER the child has formulated some conception of death and is familiar with the words representing it, the idea begins to forge habitual links with the deeper emotional life. It is as though his existent complexes annex a newly-explored territory. Where only explorers have gone before, mapping and surveying, now a constant commerce begins and the new land absorbs the interest and the passions of the old country.

Exploring and surveying demand qualities of adventure and ability which are not required of all the inhabitants of an old country. Thus the death concept now multiplies its associations with mental processes more primitive, more highly charged emotionally, than those by which the mind first made contact with the idea of death.

Analysis of the earlier stage of development led us to consider problems which have long been the province of psychologists who studied mainly the conscious processes of the mind ; this second stage is most easily described in terms of psycho-analytic theory.

V.—*The idea of death is invested with affect (emotion) through linking with (a) birth anxiety and (b) aggressive impulses.*

A. The idea of death becomes linked with birth experience mainly through three of the meanings given to death in the earlier directive exploration process. These are (i) separation, departure, disappearance ;[1] (ii) sleep ; and (iii) going into a grave, coffin, earth or water.

In the section on definitions, examples have already been given of children giving these meanings to *dead*.

EXAMPLES.   (a) *From Home Records and (b) from published literature.*

(a) *Ben, 9 : 1, and Richard, 5 : 11*

A baby had been born recently at its grandparents' house near by us, its parents' home being in the country. M. said that she wanted to go and see the baby again, but she couldn't because she had a cold, and now (about a month after the birth) she was afraid it would have gone away.

There was a moment's rather tense silence. R. looked very solemn, with big eyes. Then :

B. : What d'you mean, gone away ?

R. : What d'you mean, gone away ?

M. : Gone to its own proper home, in the country.

B. : Oh, I thought you might mean it was dead !

(b.i) *Ruth Rasmussen, aged 4 : 2*

" I once knew a hobgoblin. It had no back, and no chest, and no stomach, and no arms and no legs ; for it was dead, just like grandpa " (55.a.ii).

(b.ii) *Del, 6 plus*

" They (the roses on a rose-tree) are all withered—why ? They shouldn't die, because they are still on the tree." (53.a.i)

When the death-concept links up with birth-traces and birth-anxieties, the associations become very complex. They may be roughly set out in a table, the individual items of which will be illustrated from the records.

---

[1] For the child, absence is at first equivalent to departure, disappearance. Sully remarks that " all mothers know, when a child is asked where somebody is, who is absent, he answers ' All gone '." (66.vii). A rhythm of absence and presence is one of the earliest amusements of the baby (peep-bo), and keeps its attraction in the child's games (hide-and-seek). The whole subject has a large literature of its own.

TABLE OF ASSOCIATIONS OF DEATH WITH BIRTH

DEATH

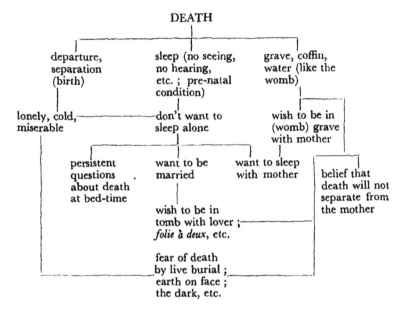

Death is equated with departure ; but to the infant the self never appears to depart. Freud has said that in the unconscious of each of us, we ourselves are immortal ; unconsciously we cannot conceive our own deaths. To the young child, death means, in the *departure* context, its mother's death, not its own. Sully found that children " dislike the idea of death as threatening to deprive them of their mother. Perhaps," he adds, " they can more readily suppose that somebody else will die than that they themselves will do so." (66.iv)

The child has a variety of ways of relieving his anxieties about the loss of his mother, which may be conveniently recorded before the anxiety-behaviour, as a safeguard for the reader against an undue access of sympathetic sentiment.

Examples of anticipatory displacement of affect.

(i) *Sonia Rasmussen, aged 4 : 7*

"Supposing I hadn't any Mummy and supposing I hadn't any Daddy, I daresay there'd be some lady or other who would give me sixpence." (55.*b*.ii)

(ii) *Ben, 8 : 8, and Richard, 5 : 6*

At lunch-time Ben said that his friend P. had told him that morning that he and his sister had been left their (dead) mother's money—"not their father !" It was in the bank, lots of it. And so now P. had the money, *and* another mother. Ben thought this a lucky thing ; on second thoughts, however, he said he would like someone he didn't like to die and leave him money. M. was not sure whether this revision of the original wish was made in regard for her presence and feelings. Richard listened without comment to all this, and then said thoughtfully to M., "I could learn to drive a car, and then you could buy a car, and you could die the next day and leave it to me."

These examples show the child's egoism in relation to death at its most perfect : the death-wish against the parents is, of course, not lacking in the home records, but examples of this charming indifference to the continued existence of the parents as persons (as distinct from the functions they fulfil) are rare.

The idea of death as being the departure of a mother from a child who needs protection, and aversion to it for this reason, become so closely associated that children will often express surprise that adults should mind their mother's death, or that a child should mind anyone else's. Thus Richard, when his grandmother was dangerously ill, found it difficult to understand his father's unhappiness, and the following conversation between himself and his mother is reported :

Richard, 5 : 11

R. : Of course Father looks like a old man, but he's not, really ; he's really quite a young man, so he still wants his mother.

M. : And you'd be sorry, too, if Granny died, wouldn't you, Richard ? Because you like going to lunch with her on Tuesdays, don't you ?

At this R. got rather worried as to whom he could go to lunch with if Granny were not available. He suggested a school friend, but evidently did not feel quite satisfied with this. Then :

R. : I've got another grandmother, haven't I ? And she could come over from (a very distant place), and when Granny dies, *she* could live at —— (Granny's house), and then I could go to lunch with her just the same.

His eyes shone with pleasure when he reached this solution of the problem. (He has never seen his other grandmother.)

Of *Judith Anson*, Richard's cousin *aged 7 : 0*, it is reported at this time that " she got very frightened—if one mother dies, her own Mummie might die, and she was often asking if I (M.) felt quite well." On another occasion :

J. : If Granny dies, I shall cry, but not for long ; I shall be unhappy because you will have no Mother ; I will be extra nice and be your Mother.

Judith is thus realizing that an adult may grieve at death, but she does this only through the identification of herself with her mother, and hence the identification of the mother with a child (her own child). As one might expect from this, she begins to think of her own death, and (aged 7 : 2) is reported as saying :

J. : Next year I shall be eight, but I might die before my birthday ; I might die before Christmas and get no presents —I might die next month—or next week—or this next minute—but I don't feel like it. I want to wait and die when you and Daddie die—it would be nice to die all together.[1]

---

[1] This remark illustrates a number of different points, as well as the immediate one. There is the wish to be with the parents in the grave and also the association of the idea of death and divisions-of-time. The matter of Judith's previous remark also illustrates points which will be more fully considered later (p. 170).

But fundamentally Judith is almost as incapable as Richard of understanding grief at any death but that of a child(self)'s mother, or at least a spouse or parent. When she was *aged 7 : 7* a little school-friend came to stay with them, because his father had died suddenly, and Judith said to her mother :

J. : Why are you sad about Mr. K. dying—he isn't your father or your husband. Geoffrey doesn't cry about it—after all, he has still got a mother.

Before the attempt is made to give a fuller picture of the development of the death-concept in connection with the birth-complex, it is necessary to turn to another equation (death equated with effect-of-old-age), which happens to be important in the development of two of the children who furnished the clearest examples in this respect. I have not records of enough children to know whether the similarity of these two boys in respect of the death-old-age equation was a necessary or a chance feature of their similar development in other ways. It was certainly not due to any contact between them or their mothers, nor was there any blood-relationship. There is four years' difference in age between the children ; they live some distance apart, and have not met more than two or three times in their lives. Their physique is quite different. They are both of them the elder of two boys.

The equation of death with effect of old age is often a very early one, directly suggested by the parents or others and readily assimilated by the child. In Ben's case we find it being suggested to him while his idea of death was still very vague. He had, however, already a keen interest in numbers, particularly through their relation to age (though not only in this relation). This interest in number *as age* was later recorded as still more marked in Ben's brother, Richard, who, from hearing it said that he *was* 5, or 6, at times almost seemed to identify himself with the number.

THE ASSOCIATION OF DEATH AND AGE

Examples.

(i) *Ben, aged 3 : 3 (in the garden with his mother)*

B. : Are you a old lady, Mother ?

M. : No, not yet.

B. : When will you be a old lady ?

M. : When I'm seventy.

B. : What will you be after you're a old lady ?

M. : I shall die, some time.

B. : And what will you be then ?

After some further talk, M. discovers that B. means, what age will she be then. She explains that one doesn't increase in age after death, but withers like flowers, or perhaps goes on a bonfire, like the withered plants.

B. : I don't want you to be a old lady, Mother.

Ben, aged 3 : 6

Ben was worrying about the end or endlessness of numbers, so M. told him there was an imaginary end called Infinity. Next morning when he woke and was babbling to himself, his father, in whose room he was sleeping, heard him say, " 'Finity !" and then, after a brief pause, " 'Finity-one, 'finity-two . . ." and so on.

Stephen, aged 4 : 10

S. was taking off his outdoor things before school, with three other children and M. present. The other children were all about a year older.

S. : My daddy has a bad cold.

Small girl : He won't get better until he's dead (frivolously).

Small boy : Stephen won't be dead for a long time.

S. (very amused and gay, in a high, squeaky, excited voice) : Edward (his brother) won't be dead for longer still. He won't be dead for a hundred years, 'cause he's only two and a half.

Small boy : Everybody'll be dead when they're a hundred.

Conversation faded out as the other children went in to class. S. turned to putting shoes on, apparently quite unmoved, as though the whole matter had slipped from his thoughts.

Stephen, aged 5 : 2

S., Edward and M. having tea in the nursery.

S. : Where's your Mummie? (He had asked this only the day before, but without any comment on the answer.)

M. : In Heaven. She died some time ago. I think she was about 70.

S. : She must have been 80 or 90.

M. : No, only 70.

S. : Well, *men* live till they're 99.

M. made no comment, and the subject changed without any further reaction from S.

Next day, tea-time :

S. : Who was my Mummie when I was one (year old) ?

M. : I was. I've always been your Mummie.

S. : When are you going to die ?

M. : Oh, I don't know. When I'm about 70 or 80 or 90.

S. : Oh ! (Pause.) When I'm grown up I shan't shave and then I shall have a beard, shan't I ? (He went on to tell a story about how he saw an old man with a long beard, and he was blowing his nose on it. He was obviously very pleased with the story. The conversation then drifted off. From a conversation on the previous day, M. gathered that he thought men grew beards when they became very old.)

THE DEATH-BIRTH COMPLEX AND ANXIETIES

In these latter entries Stephen is shown as having developed beyond the stage of being anxious about his mother's death, and is becoming anxious on his own account. While in the earlier stage, both he and Ben were very persistent in asking to have death explained to them at bed-time. Of *Ben, at the age of 4 : 0*, it is recorded :

To-night again he got very worried about when would he get up again after he was dead, and could not be satisfied with any explanation, but finally chose to postpone the matter till the next day. His last words before settling down to sleep were, " You won't forget to tell me to-morrow morning how you be dead ? Don't forget ! "

The same record continues as follows :

Since his nurse went, Ben had been sleeping with F. Now he is put in an adjoining room, since his fourth birthday. He was perfectly good, and slept well, but obviously did not like it. Three days later he said, " I wish I could be married. When can I be married ? " associating this wish with the wish to have someone to sleep with.

The talk about sleeping alone again led Ben to questions about " how you be dead " after cease-talking time, and M. said she would tell him to-morrow.

Note by M. : The postponement was not merely due to a wish to avoid a subject difficult to deal with briefly and at bed-time, but also because B. made a habit of reserving difficult questions for good-night time in the hope of luring parents into going on talking to him.

The next relevant entry is seven months later :

Ben is much less worried about death, and discusses it calmly, though with the old special interest.

More than three years elapse before the subject of death is taken up again in the same way ; then, the day following an entry of the boy's growing independence of his mother and greater pleasure in the company of his father, occurs the following :

Ben, aged 7 : 11

Ben came into M.'s bed for a minute or two before breakfast, and they talked about measles, etc.

Ben (quite happily) : I'd like to die.

M. : Why ?

B. : Because I'd like to be in the same grave as you.

This behaviour on Ben's part seems to express clearly enough the associations sleeping-alone—death ; sleeping-together—marriage ; " I don't want to sleep alone when I die ; if I could sleep with mother—not allowed now—but when I am dead it might be—then I should enjoy being dead " ; and perhaps : " after all, I did sleep with her before I was born. . . ." From such trains of thought flower certain magical and religious beliefs, discussed later.

It is not suggested that such thoughts are formulated in the mind of the child in anything like this form or logical order. It may be that links in such associative-chains are made sometimes by vaguely perceived impulses which are never presented to the mind in conceptual form, in words. On the other hand, it is evident from what these children do express, that they are actually capable of formulating such impulses in words and stating them ; adults would normally repress them. The records of the verbal behaviour of " normal " children often show how very readily they will express sentiments which the adult (and the " neurotic " child) would repress ; this ability they often combine with remarkable introspective insight. David's already quoted " I love wasps, because we kill them," is an example.[1]

The thought of the mother's death arouses a certain amount of anxiety in the child ; he is rather troubled at the thought of being lonely ; but if he has found life kind, he finds relief from this anxiety in the substitutes that reality could give him in the real event. But very soon he realizes that all men are mortal, and he is a man, so that the curse of Adam applies to himself as well. This is a very different matter. This anxiety takes many different forms. Sometimes it is apparently allayed through the equation of death with

---

[1] Certain remarks of Freud are applicable here : " We are constantly guilty of making a confusion between the phenomenon of emergence as a perception in consciousness, and the fact of belonging to a hypothetical psychical system . . . which we also call consciousness. This confusion . . . is misleading when we are dealing with the psychological system of a young child." (C.P. III, v)
(The child's mind does not present the same clear topographical divisions ; the frontiers are fluid, and the censorship is not efficiently exercised, though there is an appropriate degree of efficiency according to the child's age.)

birth. Bovet quotes Pierre Loti as saying, " My mother is the only person in the world about whom I have not experienced the feeling that death will separate us for ever " (9). A recent American research (3) brought forward this interesting contribution :

"This is the most important thing I've got to tell you (about reactions to bereavement). When I was a little kid I was terribly afraid of death, as soon as I got to know about it. I used to hope I'd be an exception to the general rule. Even in after-life I never got used to the idea, although I've cut up lots of stiffs. But do you know, when I saw my mother tucked away down there in that grave, I had no fear of death, none at all. I'd just as soon have cuddled up down there beside her as not, and since that time I haven't had the least fear of death. I remember noticing at the time that the grave wasn't so very deep, and it sort of brought her home to me. Yet when the coffin was being lowered into the grave, I wanted to holler, ' Stop ! ' "

It is clear that the incest-wish, combining with the association of grave-womb, death-sleep, has reconciled this subject to the idea of death, and has done so in his conscious thought for the first time on the actual occasion of his mother's death. Since this is all we know of the case, the supposition that the conscious fear of death, beginning in early childhood, was due to a repressed desire for death— incest—pre-natal life, can only be suggested ; the fact that the desire became conscious and the fear ceased immediately the mother was dead is, however, probably significant of this.

The naïve expression of such desires by children and by this American subject throw light on the *motif* of burial with the lover which runs so constantly through literature.[1] Romeo and Juliet meet in the tomb ; Hamlet leaps into Ophelia's grave and fights her brother there. Old ballads

[1] The subject has been studied psycho-analytically by Dr. Ernest Jones. See also Freud, *The Theme of the Three Caskets* (C.P. IV).

and fairy stories tell of unhappy true lovers buried together, and the briar that grows and twines above the grave.

> " Neither the Angels in heaven above nor the demons down under the sea
> Shall ever dissever my soul from the soul of the beautiful Annabel Lee."

—the romantic poets repeat the theme, setting the whole fantasy in twilight—Poe's " down under the sea," the " gloaming " of Keats' *La Belle Dame Sans Merci,* or the forest and night of Leconte de Lisle's *Les Elfes.* There is some deep and constant fascination in the fantasy of union in death ; and it is a desire not confined only to mature men, for we have seen that children feel it, too.[1]

B. *The idea of death is invested with affect through linking with aggressive impulses and complexes.*

In the earlier formulations of psycho-analytical theory the aggressive impulses would have been traced to the Oedipus complex, and that term might have stood for the origin of all this factor of childish aggression in relation to the development of the death-concept. More recent work, particularly Freud's theory of the death-instinct and its externalization through fusion with the erotic instincts, and Mrs. Melanie Klein's interpretations of infants' behaviour, have made the theory less simple. Aggressive impulses which are described by Dr. Ernest Jones as " grim," have been discovered in sucklings, and the development of the super-ego may originate in the rhythm of hate and remorse that fills the cradle.

[1] Two further examples have escaped from the group of those already given for children, and as most of the home record subjects are boys and these are girls, they are worth adding here.
Ruth Rasmussen, and Sonia, aged 6 : 7
R. (to her mother) : How people do love their fathers and mothers ! You mustn't die before I'm grown up.
S. (clinging close to her mother) : I shall be with you, of course. You mustn't die before I die.
Sonia, 6 : 8
You must stay with me every day, and when I die you must be in the coffin with me (to her mother) (55.*b*.iii).

If this is so, it would appear that by the time the intellectually-formulated concept of death is invaded by the affect that characterizes aggressive impulses, these impulses have already had a violent and complex history.

The death idea is brought into this system by its equation with ultimate-effect-of-aggression : it is what happens to things upon which hatred is wreaked. We have already seen that several of the school children defined death in such a way :

> Lawrence G., 5 : 2   " killed "
> Irene K., 5 : 3   " somebody's killed "
> Margaret E., 7 : 8   " somebody what's been killed "
> Joe Y., 12 : 7   " when people get murdered."

These children are expressing the attitude towards death which has been described with a wealth of detail as the attitude of many primitive peoples. Death is never a " natural " event ; it is due to the ill-will of man. Death's cause is sought only in human motive.

Thus when death is associated with aggressive impulses it is found to be rooted in human hate ; laws of nature are rejected and *lex talionis* reigns ; the two are fundamentally opposed.

The table on the next page presents some of the associations within this complex, though again the ramifications and possible combinations are far finer than can be represented in this way.

One item in this table, which might seem a matter of fantasy detail, is actually of foremost importance, namely, the place of animals in the complex.[1]

---

[1] Freud has briefly discussed the importance of animals in childish fantasy in his *Analysis of an Animal Phobia in a 5-Year-Old Boy* (C.P. IV). He points out that the child's opportunity for observing the genitals of big animals without hindrance gives the animal particular importance in the fantasy of the child. In dreams the parents are represented by large animals, siblings by small vermin, insects, etc.

It will be recalled that in classical mythology the parent gods commonly transformed themselves into animals, particularly for sexual

TABLE OF ASSOCIATIONS OF DEATH AND AGGRESSION

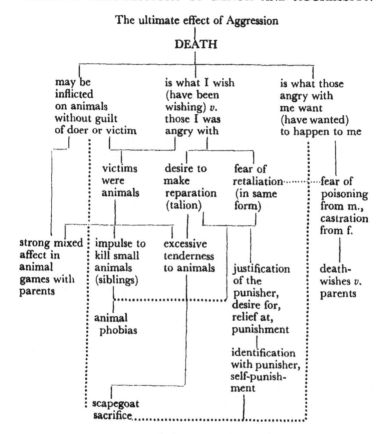

The ultimate effect of Aggression

DEATH

| may be inflicted on animals without guilt of doer or victim | is what I wish (have been wishing) v. those I was angry with | is what those angry with me want (have wanted) to happen to me |

victims were animals

desire to make reparation (talion)

fear of retaliation (in same form) ········ fear of poisoning from m., castration from f.

strong mixed affect in animal games with parents

impulse to kill small animals (siblings)

excessive tenderness to animals

justification of the punisher, desire for, relief at, punishment

death-wishes v. parents

animal phobias

identification with punisher, self-punishment

scapegoat sacrifice

ANIMALS AND THE CONCEPT OF DEATH

When we consider the place of animals, not in childish fantasy in general, but in this context in particular, we find that their great importance arises from the fact that they may be killed without social attribution of guilt. In the

practices. In fairy stories it happens that harm is done to an animal who then turns into a human being (for example, The Frog Prince, in *Grimm's Tales*), and is often mate, sib or child.

history of human culture this attitude may have been established only at the expense of severe mental conflict, which from the earliest days left a mark on religious observances.   The development from primitive totem-worship, through the animal-sacrifices of the early Semites, to the Paschal Lamb of Christianity, has been traced by Robertson Smith and his successors. Freud, in *Totem and Taboo*, led the way in linking the totem to the psychology of sex in civilized man.   The cultural environment which surrounds the civilized child is thus shown to be built on ancient fantasies of guilt and expiation.   But the association *animal—living thing—can be killed without guilt*, is not fossilized in the environment ; it is obvious.   The rabbits, which writers of romances for children write of and paint in little jackets with brass buttons and name as though they were human young, Peter Rabbit and Benjamin Bunny, these hang up dead in the shop, still with their fur coats on, easily recognizable. The child eats rabbit or chicken, and does not say grace before meat as children used to do.   People kill living things, and condone the deed, and do not suffer for it, and the thing killed does not reproach them or revenge itself.

Thus, live things which can be killed with impunity are animals, and if you have wished someone dead, and it was a human being, you are guilty, but if it was an animal you are innocent and safe.   Those against whom we have death-wishes which we cannot admit without shame and guilt are represented in our fantasies as animals.

FANTASIES INVOLVING ANIMALS AND DEATH AT EARLIER STAGES

It is not suggested that animals have no importance in children's fantasy before the death-concept is capable of finding a place there. It is obvious to all observers of child-hood that they have a great importance from very early days, and for very various reasons. But it is suggested that when death acquires deeper and wider intellectual meaning, and becomes involved in the complex of the aggressive impulses, then the animal in fantasy acquires a new importance ; it becomes the scapegoat ; it relieves the burden of guilt.[1]

Just as the animal-idea, in the earlier phases of fantasy, does not carry the same connotation as it does after death has acquired fuller meaning, so the insignia of the death event may occur in early fantasies without any of their later ("real") significance. The deeper affect with which aggressive impulses invest the death-concept flow to it *as a concept*, that is to say, an intellectually explored territory. Aggressive fantasies at earlier stages of mental development may employ the insignia of killing without involving a death-concept at all. The type of aggression which the child in this phase associates with the pre-concept of death is commonly an oral type. The wolf swallows Little Red Riding Hood's grandmother ; the witch plans to eat Hansel ; Snow White eats the poisoned apple. These activities may be fantasied without any equation of a death-concept with the oral aggression ; it is not essential to them. Freud has said that cannibalism is the sexual aim, in the oral phase.[2] Parents express their affection to children who are in this phase by getting down on all-fours, pretending to be animals, and to eat them up. Or by allowing the children to rush upon them, which they will often do growling or with open mouths, crying out " I'm a lion," etc. In courtship the statement, " I could eat you," is usually taken as a sign of amorous rather than hostile

---

[1] M. Thomas has shown that nightmares of animals are a definite stage in children's dreams, and are most common from 5 : 6–8 : 6, with maximum occurrence at 7–8 years old (71.ii).

[2] C.P. III, v. He adds that in cases where emotional disturbance has arisen " there is an anxiety belonging to this phase which manifests itself as a fear of death, and may be attached to anything that is pointed out to the child as suitable for the purpose."

intention. In simple, infantile states of mind, eating, killing and loving mingle inextricably.

Sully gives an example which shows how the child feels a need to equate " death " with oral aggression at this age. Clifford was *aged 3 : 2.*

" While he and his father were taking a walk in the country . . . they found the feathers and bones of a bird in a tiny cleft in the tree. The father thereupon " invented a story about how the unfortunate bird took shelter there, and grew " too weak to get away. The child, however, was not satisfied with this :
' P'haps a snake there, p'haps dicky bird flew there one cold winter day and snake ate it up, and then spit it out again,' and so forth. ' P'haps (he ended up) he (the bird) thought there was nothing but wind (air) there ' " (66).

Though death is commonly equated with the end-result of aggression, not all fantasies of aggression are necessarily associated with a concept of death. Swallowing may form part of a fantasied life-cycle, of which birth, or spitting out, or vomitting up again, is the next crisis, but in which death, as a specific process, has no proper part at all, having no identity in the mind which is entertaining the fantasy. In its earliest stages the concept of death may retain much of this reversability, or non-irrevocability ; and we shall see that with some children it continues to do so.

The oral aggression is a counterpart of oral erotism, and through erotism, death *qua* end-of-aggression links up with death *qua* birth-reversal.

CHILDREN'S DEATH-WISHES AND FEARS OF DEATH

Children's anger is readily expressed in hostile behaviour. The small baby's screaming and crying are a very efficient weapon, against which the parent, as enemy and victim, is often almost powerless. Action produces counter-action in kind ; fathers may be heard to say, " I could murder that child," and though it is not a matter upon which we can gather material for a statistical generalization, fathers of young infants will usually be found to agree that the reaction is normal. We may therefore be justified in classing the baby's screams as embryonic death-wishes against the parents.[1]

The child also discovers early in his life that expressions of hostility do not always bring him what he wants, but they bring counter-expressions of hostility. And expressions of hostility do not always originate with the child. His fears, therefore, are not to be invariably attributed to his own death-wishes, but may derive directly from his sense of hostility or criticism in others, which he reads in terms of his own crude impulses.

During the Story-Completion experiment many children expressed death wishes in fantasy form (see Chapter III). Some instances may now be given from the home records of death wishes or fears directly expressed.

Examples of death-wishes and fears.

Ben, aged 5 : 7
Ben called M. a silly little fool, which annoyed her. She said he was not to say that. He was annoyed with her then, and said he would put her on the bonfire and light her with fifty matches.

Aged 6 : 4
Ben (to M.) : I wish you had never been alive ! And then

---

[1] Searl suggests that the infant, by screaming, does actually destroy all that is pleasurable in his immediate experience, and also produces such exhaustion and discomfort in himself that his behaviour suggests to him (a) his own omnipotence (as effectual wisher of death) ; (b) the cruelty of " bodies," which restrain expression of emotions ; and (c) punishment in the same form as the expression of the evil wish (talion).

While there seems to be much in this argument, it appears to give insufficient weight to the ability of many babies to keep on screaming for a long time at a pressure which, from their own point of view, is well regulated. The baby who exhausts himself by screaming is not typical ; such screaming, when it arises, is likely to be due to a cause which the mother recognizes as reasonable, and she will be likely to do what she can to soothe the child. He does not destroy his world's goodness when he screams in this way.

other times I don't feel like that at all. Are you like that
with your mother ?

M. : Yes.

(Ben had been in a very bad temper before this, but after,
his bad temper went, and he immediately became very
pleasant company.)

At this time, and until he was about 7 : 6, he was unable to
sleep and would weep persistently if his mother was out late
in the evenings, and would wonder if she had been run over.
In the light of this the following entry seems relevant :

Aged 6 : 8 (at bed-time)

Ben (to M.) : I feel sort of sad and sorry about something,
sorry for you, or as though I'd done something wrong, and
I don't know why, because I haven't.

Aged 8 : 11 (one evening when F. was unexpectedly late)

Ben : D'you think he's dead ? D'you think he's had an
accident ? Are you going to ring up the police ?

Clarissa, 4 : 7[1]

C. and her mother had been talking about vets and killing
cats ; the child described how a cat was killed, and then
said :

C. : You'll die before I will. . . . I'm younger than you,
so you'll die first, won't you ?

M. : Yes.

C. (chanting happily as she went to bath) : You'll die
before me, you'll die before me.

M. went to the bathroom and kissed the child, who was
looking very happy.

C. : You *like* me, don't you ?

M. : Yes, of course I do.

C. : T.'s sister doesn't like me really. All the other
children in that form like me except J.

Note by M. : T. is Clarissa's school friend, the sister is
older than both of them. The class is the one above
Clarissa's. J., a member of this class, had shown some

[1] I am indebted for this record to a friend well skilled as a psychological observer.

hostility to her juniors, and Clarissa had made plans for killing her with bow and arrows.

Timothy, 4 : 0

(The significance of this is by no means clear ; did Timothy really consider marriage a form of punishment, or is he confusing the marriage ceremony with a funeral ceremony ? A child friend was staying with the family at the time, whose father had just died.)

Timothy had been teased by Judith ; he turned on her in anger and said : " If you are nasty to me, you will go to church and be married ! "

J. : But who shall I marry ? What do you mean ?

T. : In church, with flowers, married, and punished because you're naughty.

Judith, 6 : 11

Judith and M. were returning from escorting an aged aunt of M.'s to a bus.

J. : I think it is time aunt F. died now ; it would be better for her. May I go to her funeral when she does die ? I should like to. Will you go ?

M. : No.

J. : Well, if Granny or Uncle S. died, would you go to their funeral ?

M. : I might.

J. : Then can I go, too ?

M. : Children aren't taken to funerals ; they are such sad things. . . . You might one day watch a funeral in (the local) cemetery of someone that doesn't belong to us.

J. (emphatically and with glee) : I should love to go to Thomas O.'s funeral ; he is an *awful* little boy, and can't spell, and takes hours to write anything ; I simply hate him !

In these examples (except Timothy's) the existence of death-wishes is often very clear ; occasionally also the fear of retaliation is evident as consequence of the wish. This comes out most clearly in the Clarissa example. Ben (aged 6 : 4) shows a remarkable lack of repression of ambivalent feelings towards his mother. His behaviour indicated that his sense of guilt about his own hostility was the main cause of its persistence ; that is, the annoyance and hostility had first been aroused by objective frustration (the original record states that he had been prevented from playing with his ball while walking along the road ; it was to be kept until the cortège arrived at an open space without traffic), but the annoyance had persisted owing to the sense of guilt aroused by the hostility. The way this sense of guilt was relieved is a particularly interesting example of talion procedure : it seems as though Ben is enabled to look upon himself as nature's retaliation upon his mother for her bad wishes against her own mother ; he is instrument rather than agent. Also, of course, he has company in his guilt and in his innocence, and is at least as safe as his mother is.

CHAPTER VIII

DEATH AND LOGIC

ALREADY we have discussed under two headings how experiences and thoughts about death affect and are affected by the development of logic in the child. With the question of the association of death and the self we arrive at the heart of the problem.

To look back first at the earlier references : the subject arose with Bernard N., the boy who had lost his father, and showed obvious signs of a sense of guilt. He, it was suggested, unconsciously believed himself to be the cause of his father's death, and feared imprisonment. Later, Piaget's view was quoted, that ideas of death first bring children to conceive of chance : that is, of causation devoid of psychological motivation. The present writer suggested that this development depended upon a dominance of the positive (love) aspects of the child's main emotional attitude, and the repression of hate. For death is always possible, and if it occurs there can be no proof that it was not magically caused by human hate. But love, on the contrary, cannot for ever save the loved one, of that there is ample proof ; and so only to him in whom love is dominant does death confirm the power of impersonal causation (or natural law), and deny the potency of the individual will.

Thus the first step in the path that leads to the sovereignty of conscious Logic and Science is made through the recognition that death is inevitable for others *who are loved*. But only through the association of death with the self is the path followed to its end.

By what mental process does the child come to associate the idea of death with the idea of self? There are doubtless many different paths which link the two ideas in different minds. The path which leads many children of our culture from the one idea to the other is number as applied to age.

This association has already been illustrated in the examples previously given, particularly those of Stephen (p. 140). The same process is illustrated clearly in Rasmussen's notes on Ruth :

" *Ruth, aged 4 : 7*
    R. : Will you die, father ?
    F. : Yes, but not before I grow old.
    R. : Will you grow old ?
    F. : Yes.
    R. : Shall I grow old, too ?
(The father writes that both Ruth and Sonia at this age were extremely afraid of death. Three months later, Ruth is reported as saying, ' Every day I'm afraid of dying. . . . I wish I might never grow old, for then I'd never die, would I ? ') " (55.*a*.iii)

Through this linking of the idea of death with the idea of number, it may happen that strong affect flows into the concept of number, chronological time, ultimate beginnings and ends, and infinities of time or space. This is a subject with immense ramifications which I can only touch on with the material provided by these records : firstly with a point of curious interest. The similarity of reaction of Ben and Stephen has been noted, before and during their fifth year. In two other respects there was also a parallel : (*a*) Stephen's mother wrote of him when 4 : 10, " I think he's rather frightened of it (the idea of death), *as I used to be at the concept of Space.*" Ben's father records a conscious *horror of immense stellar distances*, which he associates with the idea of death.[1] (*b*) Ben developed a passionate interest in learning to tell the time, and could do so for many positions of the clock soon after his third birthday, and with complete efficiency a year later. For some years from that age he had a daily-tear-off calendar and rarely failed to attend to it. Number ideas were constantly in his mind ; thus, aged 3 : 1, he laid his ninepins in a row on the floor, saying, " Go to sleep, by one by one, one by one, eleven, twelve " (1 by 1 calling up the idea of 11) ; on first hearing of Jesus Christ, he said, " Was Jesus Christ very good ? " (Yes.) " Not so good as us ? " (Yes, better.) " How good—twenty ? " Stephen, during his fifth year, concentrated so much on study of the calendar that, quite by chance, I discovered he could mention at once the day of any date for months back ; he did so at the tea-table, casually, about the birthday of one of the other children present, although he had not known the date of the birthday till that moment ; and he was confirmed in what he said, and in other dates we tried him with.

The association of the idea of death and the idea of number is brought out very definitely in a report by E. Sterba of the analysis of a child who suffered from a dog-phobia :

A little girl of 7½ years, daughter of devoted parents of average intelligence and modest economic standing, brought the child to the analyst because of dog-phobia, developing two months after she had had measles, and had been given enemas. The phobia was cured after two months by allowing satisfaction for anal impulses, etc. The interesting point is that the neurosis shortly returned again, and one of its symptoms was *inability to count, and apparent loss of all knowledge of numerical relations*. . . . This, it appeared, came *from fear of death*—how soon the schoolmistress, the doctor, her mother, would die.

---

[1] Stekel writes : " I have often heard very wise and critical people say that they dare not meditate on the question of infinity or on time and space, otherwise something in the head threatened to go wrong." He discusses the subject under the heading of dread of the dead (62.i).

She told the analyst that she had a compulsive feeling to think about death and graveyards. When they spoke at school about All Souls' Day (*Lá Fête des Morts*) she was *toute bouleversée*, and could eat nothing (63).

A close linking of the idea of death with the idea of age was found in several of the school children, subjects of the tests. Two children defined death with reference to age : Pat O., " When you're old, you die," and Josie I., " When somebody's layin' dead. . . . I think she was ever so old. . . ."

More significant than these were some of the responses to story 10 (see p. 16), in which the fairy asks the child whether he would rather grow up quickly, or stay a boy (girl) for a long time, perhaps for always. Four of the boys answered that they did not wish to grow older because doing so brought death nearer.[1] Eric G. (10 : 9), for instance, said he would choose to " Stay little for a long time . . . then he would live a bit longer." Desmond I. (9 : 6) responded that the hero " said he wanted to stop a boy, so that (*i.e.*, since) as he grows older, there is less life in him." It is significant that Desmond, a boy of unusually vivid fantasy, mentioned diaries three times in different responses to the S.C. Test, and even chose to spend £100,000 on nothing but a diary.

The connection between the concept of death and the concepts of age, time, number cannot be fully studied here, but Freud's observations on the subject are too interesting to pass unnoticed. In his essay on " The Theme of the Three Caskets " he links Portia's three caskets (the third of lead), and Lear's three daughters (the third so quiet, almost

---

[1] The responses to this *Peter Pan* question demand a separate study ; it must be noted in passing, however, that no girl responded in this way, and there was a marked difference among these subjects, as to the wish to stay a child, between the boys and the girls. The responses to this question are set out according to sex and response-type in the table on the next page.

TABLE V

Showing responses to "Peter Pan" question (story 10) in relation to sex, etc.

RESPONSE	BOYS		GIRLS		TOTAL
	"N"	Clinic	"N"	Clinic	
Wish to stay a child	13	7	8	3	31
Wish to grow up quickly	21	7	23	6	57
TOTAL	34	14	31	9	88

Thus with boys, 20 : 48 (41.7 per cent) wished to stay in childhood, while with girls the ratio is 11 : 40 (27.5 per cent). If the comparatively few clinical cases are considered separately, both the ratios rise, to 50 per cent. for the boys and to 33 per cent. for the girls.

speechless), with death. The sisters are the Fates, he says, and the third is Atropos, the inevitable end. The Graces and the Hours are related to the Fates. The Hours were originally goddesses of the waters of the sky, thence of the seasons, thence of divisions of time, thence "of the law of Nature, and of the divine order of things, whereby the constant recurrence of the same things in unalterable succession in the natural world takes place." The aspect of the Hours as goddesses of destiny found expression in the Mœræ, who watch over human life.

"The implacable severity of this law, the affinity of it with death and ruin . . . its full solemnity was only perceived by mankind when he had to submit his own personality to its working.

Man struggles against recognition of subjection to death . . . ' it is only with extreme unwillingness that he gives up his claim to an exceptional position. The Goddess of Death is therefore replaced in his myth by the Goddess of Love. The Goddesses had originally been the same. And choice is substituted for necessity.'"

The child may come to the association of death with himself through the idea of old people dying—himself growing ever older—himself dying. It is a logical process, but if (as would appear from some of the records already quoted) it actually follows forms somewhat similar to those of classical logic, it is nevertheless not usually deduction proper, but what Stern has called *transduction* ; a form very commonly to be observed in the reasoning processes of the child. The major premiss is not made. The conclusion " I, too, shall die," is reached through " I, too, shall grow old," without involving the generalization, " All men grow old, all men die."

In fact, the process which Stern (64.i) observed as present in the early reasoning of children bears out Spearman's contention about the whole process of induction as actually practised ; namely, that those who use inductive processes are either basing induction on prior deduction, or else (and this he believes to occur most commonly) are reasoning not on the basis of a uniformity of natural events, but on the basis of ubiquity of causation (61.ii). So, in the child's reasoning which educes a relation between death and the self from contemplation of the consequences of growing older, the middle term is commonly not " All men are mortal " (uniformity of natural events), but " What brings Death to you will bring Death to me " (ubiquity of causation).

The conclusion is unpalatable. But the reasoning leaves a loophole. Using induction *from cause*, we state as a certainty what, after all, may be only a probability. We have stated death as a certainty for the child if it is granted to be inevitable for the adult, and if the same causation operates throughout. The next step for the child who accepts the inevitability of the adult's death is " Perhaps the same causation does not operate throughout."

(This step follows, whatever *type* of causation is envisaged. For instance, Francis, who supposes we die because Jesus kills us in the night, might take this step. But if death for the adult has not been suggested and accepted as inevitable, this step in logic does not follow.)

Now, *true* induction can prove nothing but a statistical uniformity, which still leaves infinitesimal chances ever open. So induction on the causal basis, which closed the question, is abandoned, and the child begins to ponder on the uniformity of nature (which is the basis of true deduction, and hence of true induction), not so as to accept, but in the hope of denying, the inevitability of death.

It is not suggested that the child is aware of these movements of his mind, but that children's minds may follow just this course is, I believe, made clear by the Katz's records.[1]

Theodor, aged 5 : 2

T. : Do animals come to an end, too ?

M. : Yes, animals come to an end, too. Everything that lives comes to an end.

T. : I don't want to come to an end ; I should like to live longer than anybody on earth.

M. : You need never die ; you can live for ever.

Aged 5 : 4

T. : Was God born ?

M. : God wasn't born and God doesn't die. . . .

T. : If God doesn't die, then all men won't die.

M. : I'll tell you all about that when you are bigger.

T. : You shouldn't say things like that ; it's rude.

Theodor, on the basis of a perceived non-uniformity in

---

[1] (Katz reference, 35.iii.) It may be suggested in this connection that possibly the analyst who treated the case recorded on p. 157 missed an underlying cause in both onsets of the neurosis ; in the dog-phobia, the connection of animal and death ideas, and in the number-difficulty, the application of death to the self. This application is obscured in the French translation, but the German for *All* Souls' Day corresponds more to the English than the French, and gives the clue to why the child was " *toute bouleversée* " particularly then, and went to meet, by starvation, the death she feared. Her desire (for food) failed, " because man goeth to his long home."

M

supposed natural events, is moved to deny the validity of a law which, as he well perceives, can only be securely founded on such an absolute uniformity. He rightly feels it " rude " when the maturity of his intelligence is impugned after such an intellectual achievement. For although his argument reproduces traditional religious arguments too closely to be imagined unsuggested, the logical sequence is obviously a result of his own individual impulse.

Further than this, in the positive development of logic in the individual child, our present material does not go. But later (in Chapter X) we shall return to these records of Theodor, and to others, which show with what strong affect children will attempt to refuse mental admission to logic's findings when it brings together the self and death.

CHAPTER IX

DEATH AND MAGIC

GENERAL ASPECTS OF CHILDREN'S MAGICAL THOUGHT

THE magical thoughts that children express, and the magical rites they act, flow from mental attitudes that condition and explain them. This is particularly true of the child in civilized cultures, because his magic is sporadic and spontaneous : it does not grow in harmony with the social environment, as primitive magic does ; it seldom crystallizes into an organized system of thought and custom. Its *raison d'être* is to be found in the individual child's personal need.

Although adults continue to think magically, some seldom (in thoughts which enter consciousness), some consciously and openly throughout their lives, yet the magical thoughts and behaviour of children tend to strike every adult with a shock of surprise. For this reason they are often noted by the observer who has no psychological training ; noted, that is to say, without context, and without attempt to appreciate their significance in the system in which they belong. They are noted merely for their bizarre quality, set against the background of what to them is foreign, namely, the attitude of thought which the adult considers normal.

It would be comparatively simple to collect in this way children's sayings and practices of a magical colour, bearing on the concept of death, but such a collection could claim little value without psychological interpretation. On the other hand, this particular aspect of magical thought in children of civilized culture has been only slightly treated in some of the most penetrating studies of children's magical thought, mainly because of difficulties inherent in the subject matter. Hence publication of data in itself has a certain value, apart from the evaluation and interpretation that may accompany it. For this reason, records will be quoted at some length, rather than merely referred to in illustration of argument.

DEFINITION OF MAGIC

Professor Piaget's work, which is the classical corpus for this subject of children's magical thought, has defined *Magic* on the basis of Lévy-Bruhl's theories, as *the use of participation to modify reality ;* and *Participation* he defines as *a primitive idea of a relationship between two things or beings regarded as identical or mutually influential, when there is no direct contact or intelligible causal connection between them* (53.*c*.i).[1]

This definition is useful, but it raises difficulties because it begs the question of what is intelligible and what is causal. Dr. Ruth Benedict defines *Magic* as *setting a pattern for the desired event.* Systems of thought are not, of course, to be confined in sentences, and definitions of them are only useful counters. One a little different from either of these seems to suit the present research better, and to be equally valid. *Magic,* let us say, is *behaviour which implies the belief that things happen as they are thought, wished, or acted.*[2]

The word " as " is here used with all its variety of meaning ; and its different meanings connote different types of magic. It may mean " in the way that," and refer to a magic of analogy ; it may mean " because," and refer to the magic of thought's effectiveness, (though in that case " acted " has a limited, dramatic meaning) ; it may mean

---

[1] Piaget states that in making use of L-B.'s definition, " absolutely no identity is implied between the child's magic and the magic of the primitive."

[2] The three activities might all be included under a single word, if there existed a word to cover the whole of mentally motivated activity.

" while," and refer to a magic of simultaneity, and it may include similarity apparent in exact reversal or negation. Most commonly magical behaviour will show a combination of at least two of these types.

Magical thought does not preclude logic or science. Things do happen as they are thought, if we think rightly. Roughly we may say that here the main difference is not ultimately in the method, but in the attitude the subject takes towards the method—towards his thinking. Science treats the thought as a hypothesis, to be tested under conditions sufficiently various or controlled to cheat the personal element out of the equation. The scientist attempts to put the " happening " in control of the situation ; he says, *Let us think how things happen.* The magician says, *Things happen as we think.*[1] In societies based on magic, the successful magician is actually very often a scientist ; in societies based on science, the scientist is perhaps occasionally a magician.

Logic may be used to drive home a magical premiss as surely as an empirically sound one. For this reason, to make a contrast between phases of children's thought as magical or logical may, I believe, produce more difficulties than it solves. To take an example from the Katz records : the little boy, Julius, was one day stroking his father's hand when by mistake he scratched it. Then he said that the scratch was done by the air. Then, to his father :

J. : Is the air wicked ?
F. : No, the air is not wicked.
J. : But why did it scratch with its finger ?

What are the mental processes behind this dialogue ?

---

[1] It is not intended to suggest that the " magician " would ever make such a statement. Magic is an attitude of mind which precedes any formulation of itself, and may precede the conception of " thinking " as distinct from " happening."

We may conceive them as follows : " I scratched—it's wicked to scratch—I didn't mean to do it, I wish I hadn't done it—so I didn't do it (magic)—but it was done—by someone, something—there is nothing but air—the air did it (conclusion)—the air is wicked (corollary)."

There are, perhaps, certain omissions from the train of thought as given above. Julius may have first thought, " It's wicked for *a boy* to scratch *his father*," and repressed the most highly affective part of his thought. Thus he repressed the personal motive, and this repressed factor has determined the magical factor : " air " is substituted for " boy." But in the train of thought as given above, it will be seen that only the one magical link is needed, and with that one link one can come to a logical conclusion such as Julius reaches.

Now, Julius is no doubt aware that he has reached a *reductio ad absurdum*, but the logic and the actual conclusion are quite secondary considerations. The point is, is the scratcher of the finger wicked ? His father says, No, the air is not wicked. This obviously makes things much easier. Fathers can be scratched without guilt. And if the air is not wicked, the boy, whose intentions also were innocent, may not be wicked either. " But why did the air scratch *with its finger ?* " Julius then asks, showing that he is already half way to accepting reality, now that the magical agent has done its work. And if now he is answered, " But it didn't," he will be able to agree. The magic was a mechanism by which he managed to detach guilt from his action. When that is done he can look reality in the face again. He *projected* the guilt and the action into " happenings," external things, and now, having had them pronounced innocent and the guilt wiped away, he will be able to acknowledge the act again as his own.[1]

Julius wanted to project the sense of guilt from himself, so

---

[1] If the child were answered, " But you know it didn't," his attention would be turned to the validity of the mechanism, and anxiety would probably be increased rather than diminished.

he projected it into Nature. But it may happen (perhaps partly as an after-effect of the use of this mechanism) that we fear the unknown forces of nature, as agents, more than we fear our fellow-men. Then we have an interest in introjecting into humanity all causation. Fear is found capable of control, if the event arises from a source so familiar as psychological motivation ; statistical causality (" Fate ") is blind. It arouses something of the same panic horror as the blind men who are so uncannily efficient in H. G. Wells's story, *The Country of the Blind.* The most familiar kind of psychological motivation is that to which the self's own body acts as agent ; introjecting the evil cause into the self is a reaction to maximal sense of discomfort or anxiety at the powers of the unknown, Fate.

MAGICAL THINKING AND THE CHILD'S CONCEPTION OF DEATH

Morgenstern, in a psycho-analytical study of magical thinking in the child, stated that any one of life's problems might come within the range of the child's magical thinking, but that it occurs above all in connection with problems of birth and death.

Among the various magical ideas which children express about death one may discover a certain order. When the death-concept is equated with one of the ideas which link it with the complex of birth (*i.e.*, separation, the tomb, sleep), there results a belief that the actual pattern of life in time will be symmetrical, with a symmetry suggested by the common aspects of birth and death as union with and separation from the mother (who is also regarded unconsciously as the wife). Many similarities can be found between the life before birth and the life after death : we begin and we end in nothingness and mystery and dispersed elements—we begin helpless and we end helpless. " Our little life is rounded with a sleep." Magical thinking converts analogies into similarities and similarities into identities : the English language popularly uses *like* for *as* : things happen in the same way as they are thought (and wished) ; the things that happen are like things that are thought (wished) : the thing that happens *is* the thing that was wished ; birth and death are identical. We may find examples of this thought-train at different stages : sometimes the child will but reach the stage of apprehending a symmetry ; sometimes he will suggest that death is a pre-natal life.

But when the death-concept is equated with an idea which connects it with the aggressive complex, the magic seems to depend more on psychological motivation as cause (although analogy may also have a place). To feel angry with X. is to want to kill X., and the want is causative ; I am causing the death of X. by wanting it ; I am a murderer. If X. is angry with me, he is killing me. If the aggressive wish is particularized in some other way (orally, anally, genitally) then the retaliation will be similarly particularized, symbolically.

Naturally the mental processes are never so simple as this ; and there is an obvious omission that is especially important. The essence of the whole process is, that I and X. participate in each other's mental existence. The I is not only himself ; he is X. as well ; he has identified himself with X. (to some extent *whoever X. may be*). " I " is his own father, he is his own mother, but further, he is human, *nihil humanum sibi alienum est;* he is X. and feels injured and aggrieved in his own person at his own aggression.

We have seen in Bernard's case that if X. really dies, the I fears imprisonment, or some other retaliation, with extreme vividness, and may be preoccupied with the idea of guilt almost obsessionally. It must be stressed that Bernard was an apparently normal little boy, holding his own in his ordinary school class, and able to exercise his intelligence (otherwise) in an absolutely normal way. He was not " clinical material."

Other characteristics differentiating the type of magic flowing from the birth and aggression complexes will be noted later ; they can be best studied from concrete examples.

Examples of magical thinking : birth-death symmetry.

Richard, aged 3 : 11
Richard remarked when M. was undressing him for his bath, that when he is a man, M. will be a little boy or girl, and he (R.) will bath her and put her to bed.

Richard, aged 4 : 4
Richard wanted to know where babies come from : on being told, he said, would he go back inside M. when he was five ? (*i.e.,* on his next birthday).

Francis, aged 5 : 1
Francis saw a coffin being carried into a house, and arrived for his bath full of excitement. There was some conversation about the coffin, why it had to be nailed down, etc. Then :

F. : Of course the person who went away (*i.e.,* in the coffin) will become a baby.

M. : What makes you think so ?

F. : Of course he will, won't he ?

M. : I don't know.

F. : When John (F.'s baby brother) was born, someone must have died.

All this was said in a tone of conviction, as if there were no doubt about it. The conversation then changed to the subject of the dripping taps. He was having his bath while the recorded incident took place.

The first belief expressed above is not properly a belief about death, but it is a belief about the end of life. Although it is the only instance of its kind among these subjects, such beliefs of children have frequently been referred to in psychological literature. Sully gave instances of it (66.vi), and Dr. Ernest Jones studied it in an essay, *The Significance of the Grandfather*.[1]

" With many children (writes Dr. Jones) there is a lively desire to become the parents of their own parents, and they may even entertain the fantastic belief that just in proportion as they grow bigger, so will their parents grow smaller, till in time the present position of affairs will be completely reversed. This curious construction of the imagination, which is probably one of the sources of the belief in reincarnation, is evidently closely connected with incestuous wishes, since it is an exaggerated form of the commoner desire to be one's own father. It also subserves a hostile attitude towards the parents, and gratifies the wish to change the actual situation in such a way that the child is in a position to order those about who now order him."
(34.*b*)

" There are several component parts of the phantasy—the gradual reversal in size, the extension of the belief that the child is in imagination the actual parent of its parent—*i.e.*, equivalent to its own grandfather—and the consequences of the phantasy in adult life, especially as regards the attitude to children and the belief in reincarnation. . . . Our children, just like adult savages, imagine that when an old person dies he will shortly reappear as a new-born child."
(34.*c*)

As Dr. Jones points out, the idea of the reversal of parts between child and parent—the arc-like symmetry, or serial-arc conception of the life-process—is closely allied to the idea of reincarnation. The ideas of Francis may easily be seen as a development of the ideas of Richard.

---

[1] Dr. Jones apparently attached some significance to the grandparent being male, but in the example given above (Richard), and in that on p. 138 (Judith), the child imagined itself the *mother* of its mother (*i.e.*, the grandmother of itself), not the (grand)father. Does the incestuous-wish component of the fantasy survive this transposition, irrespective of the homosexuality at which we now arrive?

Both appear to derive from an equation of birth and end-of-life.[1]

The arc-symmetry conception of life is a development prior to the idea of reincarnation (although some of the children who express the latter idea are chronologically younger). Dr. Susan Isaacs reports the case of a little girl with whom the circle was, in imagination, completed within the same family :

" Z., *aged 5,* asked if an aunt was dead ; her mother asked her what happened to people when dead.

Z. : They go back into their Mummie's tummy and become a teeny-weeny baby again." (33.*b*.i)

Examples of ideas of reincarnation.

First will be given a series of reincarnation ideas as they were expressed by one subject over a considerable period of time. The first instance is not a reincarnation idea, but it helps to explain how that idea arose. This item itself follows on that given on p. 140, where the mother likened human life and death to that of flowers.

Ben, aged 3 : 4

While Ben and M. were gardening, a friend stopped at the gate to talk to them. After she went on :

Ben : Does Mrs. X. (next-door neighbour) know Margery ?

M. : No, I know her because I was at school with her.

---

[1] For this reason it is difficult to understand why Hocart, describing those primitive death-customs which involve a reversal of every life-custom, classes them as *Death Customs not derivable from Birth,* and leaves them in a limbo of their own (28). These inversions take all kinds of forms :

" returning in inverse order from the burial ground . . . backward speech, inverting weapons, and the like. The living are by inversion imitating the dead, among whom everything is inverted : our day is their night. . . . It seems that under the earth, everything is upside down."

One may compare the position of the child in the womb, who also is " upside down."

B. : Where were I, then ?

M. : You weren't anywhere at all.

B. : Yes, I were inside you.

M. : No, I don't think you were anywhere.

B. : I were under your feet.

Note by M. : Ben was quite familiar with the idea of gestation. The conversation was not a very serious one, but B. seems to have had in mind a process of growing up from a root, like the plants we were dealing with at the time.

Aged 3 : 4

Ben, on being told how the same plants come up again in the spring, after being invisible above ground in the winter, asks when should we all be dead and gone, and then come back again.

Aged 4 : 10

Ben invented and typed the following story, being told which letters would be needed for the words he said he wanted :

" A boy once was very bad for always and always and always, he was the king's boy, and the queen's boy, and when he was born again he was very good. It was me, (Ben), and it was Mrs. (Clement)'s boy."

Aged 5 : 9

Ben heard for the first time about evolution and the descent of man.

Aged 6 : 7

Ben was doing up his shoes. M. sneezed.

B. : Funny how you can't remember your life before at all.

M. : Yes. What made you think of that ?

B. : Because you can't imitate a hitchoo (sneeze).[1]

---

[1] From the point of view of comparison of child and primitive psychology this is the most striking contribution of all the home records, and the one least easily explained. Frazer (*The Belief in Immortality and the Worship of the Dead*, p. 193–4) writes : " Sneezing is a sign that the soul has returned to the body, and if a man does not sneeze for many weeks together, his friends look on it as a very grave symptom ; his soul, they imagine, must be a very long way off." Ben's thought also has affinities with Platonism.

Ben, 9 : 0 ; Judith, 7 : 0

Judith came to spend the day with Ben. There was talk
about (their grandmother) at lunch-time (who was seriously
ill). Ben referred to being born again, in a thousand years.
Judith said, " That would be nice," but Ben really seemed
to believe it.

Ben, 9 : 2 ; Richard, 6 : 1 (having breakfast with F.)

B. (to F.) : Would you like to be H. ? (a friend of F.'s
who died when Ben was a baby).

F. : No ; I don't specially want to be dead . . . but if
I were in heaven, I might be going to cricket matches every
day.

B. : Oh, no, you would be in church every day ; Heaven
is very religious. . . . I expect Richard Cœur-de-Lion is
soon going to be born again. . . . Mother says you get
born again about every thousand years. . . .(1)

F. : Why do you have to wait so long ? Why shouldn't
you be born again the year after you died ?

B. : Oh, no ; because then you'd be able to remember
everything that happened before. . . . I can remember you
in my last life, Richard. Can you remember me ?

R. : Yes, I can remember you.

. . . . . .

B. : Perhaps I was Richard Cœur-de-Lion. . . .

R. : Then I was Ben Cœur-de-Lion !

F. (to Richard, whose suggestion has been scoffed at by
Ben) : You might have been St. Benedict.

B. : Yes, I was Richard Cœur-de-Lion, and before that
I was Julius Cæsar, and before that Caractacus, and before
that a monkey, and before that a crab, and before that a
tiny little insect, and before that I was in the sun ; a great
big tree growing in the sun !

(1) *Note by M. :* This was probably Ben's conclusion from
some non-committal answer to a proposition of his own.

(Richard never has spontaneous reincarnation ideas, but
occasionally falls in with Ben's. His own view is that
" when you are dead, you stay dead." When Ben said that

in a next life Richard might be " a tree or a bird," Richard went on " or part of the table, or this piano.")

Ben, aged 8 : 9, and again 9 : 3, said he would rather be buried than burned, after death, and the latter time explicitly said it was because then he could be born again.

Now to leave Ben and turn to an entry of *Catherine Holland, aged 9 : 0.*

Catherine, returning from an afternoon walk with M., Susanna aged 6 : 10, and baby John, asked, apparently *à propos* of nothing :

" What happens to people when they are dead ? Are they eaten by worms ? Or do they go and dance about in heaven ? I'll tell you all about it when I'm born again !— Are you born again ? "

M. said some people said so. The subject was then dropped. The tone was flippant until the last four words.

————

The magical beliefs which children express as theirs appear sometimes to be surprisingly spontaneous (as, for instance, Ben's remark about the sneeze), but very frequently it may be found, where full records are kept from an early age, that some statement of an adult has given the child a first suggestion, which he has accepted and developed. In such a case, the assimilated creed or theory may nevertheless be accepted as an authentic part of the child's own thought. This applies no less to traditional religious teachings which the child absorbs, and which function thereafter as mental processes of his own personality. Instances of this have already been given under other heads. Few children in England fail to be provided with the association of death—heaven—sky. The home records, however, give no instance of a complete assimilation of this teaching. Richard, who had no leanings towards reincarnation, was interested in Heaven from his fourth year, when imbued, rather unsystematically, with orthodox Church of England views, but his reactions became later definitely negative :

Richard, aged 6 : 6 (lunching alone with M.)

R. : Miss S. (his school teacher) says there is a God. But I don't believe there is.

M. : Don't you, Richard ?

R. : No. Because nobody's ever seen Him. So how can they know He's there ?

M. : Did you tell Miss S. ?

R. : No. But I told the other children.

(Here M. lost some remarks, owing to the business of recording.)

R. : Miss S. says there must be a God. Because He made the world. But I don't think the world was *made*. I think it just *came*. . . . Perhaps a pilot would know. Because He's up in the air (*i.e.*, God ; the pilot, to Richard, means always an aeroplane-pilot).

M. : I don't think He's up in the air.

R. : Up in Heaven—only we've never seen Him on the ground, God.

Richard's location of Heaven as up in the air (which is, of course, very common, being suggested by the terms of the Christian tradition) may have been strengthened by some remarks of Ben on the subject over a year before. The two brothers were playing with another boy when the following conversation took place (taken down simultaneously by M., whose presence the children seemed to have forgotten) :

Ben, aged 8 : 6 ; Robert, aged about 7 : 6 ; Richard, aged 5 : 4

(The children saw a picture of " Goosey, goosey gander," and chanted the rhyme through. Then :)

Ben : And *you* don't say *your* prayers, Richard !

Richard : I don't know what it means.

Ben : A thing you say to God.

Robert : What you say to God at night, isn't it, Ben ?

Richard : But I don't know what God is ! (distressed).

Ben : God's a thing that isn't really (laughing). At least, that's what I think, only I pray to Him. A kind of imaginary thing that floats about in the air. At least, that's what I think.

It would, however, lead too far away from the subject of death, to show by what logical paths Ben had come to this theological position.

None of these children are recorded as having mentioned Hell in connection with death, but Ben, 8 : 11 and 9 : 0, wondered whether God would be nasty to him when he went to Heaven, or angry with him because he " didn't like the Bible."

REINCARNATION WITHIN THE FAMILY

Francis thought that when his baby brother John was born someone must have died. Z. (p. 171) thought the dead person went into the mother's " tummy " and became a baby again. Ben, we find, from the following example, thinks that the father may die in the act of giving life.

Ben, 8 : 10, and Richard, 5 : 8 (having tea with M.)

We were talking about the youngest king ever, and Richard was much interested and amused when Ben and M. spoke of the King of Spain who was king before he was born. Ben then showed that he thought the father died as a result of begetting the child. M. said she did not think the two things would be connected with each other. Ben said, " But mothers sometimes die when the children are born." M. said again that she did not think anyone ever died as a result of " making a baby begin." Ben said he thought something might come out of the father's inside that oughtn't to, and so he might die.

Ben does not suggest that the child may reincarnate the father. But the particular case which suggested to him that the father lost his life in giving life to the child is the case of a king, and of a child who becomes king in his father's place.

A similar idea was of very great importance (according to a recent study) in the life of Gustav Fechner, whose father had a posthumous child. Fechner's father died, after a long illness, when the boy was five years old.

"The youngest daughter of the family was born just one day after the father's death, and the child Gustav interpreted this coincidence as meaning that the father had died in giving another life, associating the event with a strong feeling of guilt" (27).

We have here an idea which spans the division between the birth and aggression associations of death. The examples previously given, of magical conceptions of death, are ideas of analogy of death with birth ; ideas of a symmetrical or serial-symmetrical pattern of existence ; ideas in which a sense of guilt does not appear to play a part. A sense of rivalry between the child and the father for the body of the mother does not become apparent in these preceding examples. The thinker seems to be as little preoccupied with the claims of the father as the child in the womb or the small nursling would be. But when birth involves the father's death, incarnation and reincarnation become guilty.

MAGIC AND THE AGGRESSIVE IMPULSES

If the findings would fit into a neat scheme, one would begin here a new section, showing the magical beliefs parallel to those of reversal of the generations and of reincarnation, which accompany the association of the death idea with the aggressive impulses. But the results of these different associations are not parallel in behaviour and belief. The fantasies which arise in connection with aggressive impulses do not become beliefs. They are not, in the child, repressed into the unconscious mental system as they are in an adult. They can become, in a sense, conscious ; they can be put into words and perceived. But they are not believed in as true (or even provisionally true hypotheses), which organize reality into an explanation of life as it is. They are not recognized to be on the same plane as beliefs ; they are fancies.

N

One example will make the difference clear. On a summer holiday, it is recorded, Ben (aged 8 : 6) and his mother felt a good deal of friction in their relationships. One day, however, they went for a long and friendly walk alone together, and when they sat down to rest far away from everyone else, Ben remarked, thoughtfully and confidentially, " I sometimes think you are a witch, and don't like me at all, really, and will put poison in my food."

Now it is quite possible that Ben holds his reincarnation theories as somewhat hypothetical ; but his preference for burial over cremation is a real preference, on which he would be prepared to act without any sense of irrationality. This idea of his mother poisoning him, however, is one on which he never showed the slightest tendency to act, though it is an actual motivation in the case of many neurotic children.

We may therefore distinguish three types of magical idea as expressed by children :

(1) Ideas which relieve intellectual tension, but may involve no further degree of essential affect. They become conscious as belief or hypothesis.

(2) Ideas which derive from the love-aspect of an ambivalent relationship and ignore rivalry. These ideas may also become in every sense conscious, as belief or hypothesis.

(3) Ideas which derive from erotism, complicated by rivalry and/or by the conflicts of ambivalence. These ideas become in the " normal " child embryonically (as it were) unconscious. That is, they may be expressed verbally, but they will not be looked upon as true beliefs or hypotheses ; they will be expressed as fantasy, either in words, movements or play.

The first group scarcely concerns us here, since the idea of death invariably involves essential affect after the earlier (intellectual exploration) stage. Many of the magical beliefs associating death with birth or pre-natal life belong to the second group. They may become conscious as belief or hypothesis, and have been illustrated by the examples already given in this chapter. But with the third group we turn away from the whole realm of belief and " rational " hypothesis, to the realm of fantasy : fantasy such as we have already studied in Chapter III. Bernard's obsession with the idea of imprisonment and guilt has already made clear how the child, like primitive man, may feel that where there is death there is a murderer, and that the child, who must necessarily be rival to the father or siblings for the mother's body, time, and attention, must be that murderer. Although he has six siblings, Bernard could scarcely feel more keenly his own guilt for his father's death.

MAGICAL PRACTICES ARISING FROM ANXIETIES ABOUT DEATH

The home records tell of behaviour on the part of some of these children which, although we can scarcely say it shows any but the mildest anxiety, or any but the most rudimentary magic, yet parallels examples given elsewhere which are more explicit in both these respects. Thus Ben, who associated the idea of death with age when he was three years old, amused himself, but also sometimes worried himself, by imagining numbers never stopping (" 'finity-one, 'finity-two ") ; Stephen decided not to shave when he grew up because men live to be older than women, and old men have beards ; Ben refused to have any contact with death, and would not let flowers wither in his hand ; Catherine thought that to kiss a dead body was disgusting.

Behind the reactions of Ben and Catherine evidently lie mental processes which have led, in social psychology, to an immense edifice of belief and ritual, symbolized by the word " sacred " and its etymological connections. The idea of the sacred includes that of the untouchable as unclean, and as holy, and as a part of the body guarding sexual organs, and it is constantly associated with a certain mental attitude to the bodies of the dead, in which sympathetic magic undoubtedly plays a part.

The close association which may grow up between the ideas of death and of number is illustrated in several of the examples of magical thinking given by Professor Piaget (*The Child's Conception of the World*). The following is one of these :

" Every evening, from about the age of 6 to 8, I was terrified by the idea of not waking up in the morning. I used to feel my heart beating and would try, by placing my hand on the chest, to feel if it was stopping. It was undoubtedly in this way that I started counting to reassure myself. I counted very quickly between each beat and if I could succeed in passing a certain number before a particular beat or in making the beats correspond with even or with uneven numbers, etc., I felt reassured. I have forgotten the details, but I can remember the following very clearly. At regular intervals, from the pipes of the radiator in my room, would come a sudden, deep, rattling sound, which often used to make me jump. I used to use this as a proof of whether I should die or not ; I would count very fast between one rattle and the next, and, if I passed a certain number, I was saved. I used the same method to know whether my father, who slept in the next room, was on the point of death or not " (53.*c*.iii).

The following incident, which Piaget quotes from Flournoy, is provided by a woman :

" One of my most distant memories relates to my mother. She was very ill and had been in bed several weeks, and a servant had told me she would die in a few days. I must have been about 4 or 5 years old. My most treasured possession was a little brown wooden horse, covered with ' real hair.' . . . A curious thought came into my head : I must give up my horse in order to make my mother better. It was more than I could do at once and cost me the greatest pain. I started by throwing the saddle and bridle into the fire, thinking that ' when it's very ugly, I shall be able to keep it.' I can't remember exactly what happened. But I know that in the greatest distress I ended by smashing my horse to bits, and that on seeing my mother up, a few days later, I was convinced that it was my sacrifice that had mysteriously cured her and this conviction lasted for a long while " (53.c.ii).

The first instance shows again the close association that may grow up between the ideas of death and number. In the second case it may be supposed that an unformulated sense of guilt had urged the child to make reparation for a death-wish ; certainly she has the impression that her actions influence Death ; if she can prove that she would give her most cherished possession rather than have her mother die, then her benevolence will save her mother's life. The fact that the matter requires painful and tangible proof suggests that a sense of ambivalance was a motivating factor ; the fact that the victim was a loved *animal* suggests that upon this toy had been showered some of the love which was felt as due to the mother, and also that the scapegoat of the crisis had played a part of dual-identification with both the loved and hated aspects of the parent.

CHAPTER X

In the children who were subjects of this research, anxiety about death appeared to occur in two different forms, one chronic and the other critical. The chronic form of death anxiety appears to be a reaction from aggressive impulses and to begin before there is a clear conception of death. It has its individual crises (as when a member of the family dies or is seriously ill), and it may take many forms, as for instance, a fear of imprisonment because of supposed death-guiltiness, or a fear of one's own death because of supposed or actual aggression-guiltiness, or a fear of the actual death of a person wished dead, combined with a fear of acute consequent remorse and loneliness for the self. Such anxiety is chronic, however, in that it may occur in some form at any stage in the life of a " normal " person.

The critical anxiety observed in children, on the other hand, tends to occur at a definite stage of development ; that is, when death, given a meaning of B–E category, first comes into mental association with the idea of the self, when the self-idea has been understood or differentiated to a corresponding degree. It then appears as though the mechanisms used by the ego to defend itself against the more primitive death anxiety arising from id-impulses are of no avail when it is called upon to deal with the more objective kind of anxiety which arises later. The earlier type of anxiety may be allayed by projection of guilt (as with Julius Katz), or introjection of it (as with Bernard N.). Julius *projected* the bad action from himself on to the neutral elements ; he then secured from the victim an exoneration of the elements (the air is not wicked) ; and then (as I have suggested) he was prepared to reappropriate the action, and to accept reality. Bernard *introjected* the agent of death into himself, against all the evidence of the senses or the circumstances. It has been suggested that his unconscious motive (and perhaps also the unconscious motive of primitive people) in doing this is inability to tolerate the notion of a blind, impersonal Fate ; that all magical ideas of this kind (that is, all ideas of participation which put causal responsibility exclusively on human factors) originate in a rejection of, or inability to apprehend, impersonal causation—a rejection which may be a form of repression, and which in primitive society becomes the social convention and tradition.

Both these mechanisms help the individual to reconcile himself to the death or injury of others. But when the course of noetic synthesis through maturation brings death into relation with the self, they are of little use to the civilized child. As we have already seen from the records, some children at this stage are reconciled to a sufficient degree of reality for their purposes by developing the belief in reincarnation, which they can do with the less conflict because it is mainly based on a love-aspect of an erotic relationship. There are others whose development does not follow these lines. They may, at the stage of association of death with the self, go through a period of anxiety, which in some cases will be acute and manifest. Theodor Katz[1] and Richard Clement appear to have gone through this unhappy experience, but it does not occur in the records of any

---

[1] Above, p. 161. Reference No. 48. Dr. Katz writes, p. 251 : " Our children spoke quite often about murder and shooting . . . but a presentment of the tragedy behind death is only to be seen in one conversation with Theodor (No. 33). . . . From his attitude and tone of voice, rather than from the actual formulation of the words, it was clear that the child had been touched by the seriousness of the problem of death."

" normal " child in so extreme a form as in a neurotic case
reported by a psycho-analyst, as follows :

"La première notion de la mort peut déclencher chez
l'enfant des réactions affectives très intenses. Une petite
fille de quatre ans pleura pendant 24 heures, quand elle
apprit que tous les êtres vivants meurent. Sa mère ne put
la calmer par aucun autre moyen que par la promesse
solennelle qu'elle, la petite fille, ne mourrait jamais. Cette
même fillette a eu, à l'age de quinze ans, une toux hystérique
d'une durée très longue et d'une acuité excessive. L'analyse
de ce cas démontra qu'il s'agissait d'un acte d'autopunition
pour des désirs inconscients de mort envers sa mère, sa sœur
et ses frères. Elle se voyait atteinte de tuberculose et
mourante. . . ." (51.i).

It may be asked, what is the *type* of this anxiety. In terms
of the classification which Anna Freud has made familiar,
does it derive from the ego's fear of being overwhelmed by
id-impulses directly ; or from the ego's fear of the severity of
its own ideals, its conscience or super-ego ; or from fear of
an external, objective danger ; or from conflict of impulses ?
The answer appears to be certainly the third form ; this is
an objective fear, but it is of a secondary nature. All fear
of external danger presumably must operate through
secondary mental processes—that is to say, according to a
reality principle as well as a pleasure-pain principle. The
anxiety about death, however, is secondary in still a further
degree ; that is to say, it is a primary fear (as of loneliness in
babyhood or possibly the original anxiety of birth itself)
reactivated not merely (or rather, not usually) through
percepts, but through the ideational associations which can
only be built up above the perceptual level.

To return to the actual cases : the little French girl is
deeply affected at hearing that *all* men are mortal, and her
anxiety is only relieved by simple absolute negation of what
she had already received as reality ; negation, at least in so

far as that reality affects her personally. Exactly such an assurance we have already observed as being given to little Theodor by his mother.

A similar example is to be found in the home records :

Richard, aged 5 : 1
Once or twice lately, at bath-time, R. has begun to get whimpering and miserable about dying. Yesterday he played with the possibility of never dying, living to a thousand, etc., as he swam up and down in his bath. But to-day :
R. : I might be alone when I die. Will you be with me ?
. . . But I don't want to be dead, ever ; I don't want to die.
This raised difficulties, because a day or two before his trouble had seemed to be that he did not know how to die ; he seemed to be worried mainly about his inefficiency, and M. had told him he need not worry, because she would die first, and he could see what it was like—this seemed to satisfy him at the time. However, M. now assured him that she would be with him when he died. Then :
M. : But you won't die for a long time, Richard. You won't die till after you understand about it.
At this a smile gradually broke over his very serious, unhappy face, and he said : That's all right. I've been worried, and now I can get happy. (He jumped about on the bath-mat, and sang a little with relief.)
A few minutes later :
R. : I wish I could dream in the day-time.
M. : What would you like to dream about ?
R. : About going shopping and buying things.

Taking these three examples together—of the little French girl, Theodor and Richard—we may observe two significant things which they all have in common : (1) the mothers' reactions ; (2) that the children are all concerned to deny something they have already conceived.

The mothers assured the children that they would not die (for the question of postponement until there was understanding is practically equivalent to this). The outsider might be inclined to deprecate this behaviour, or even to censure it. And it is possible that the mothers would, perhaps somewhat hesitatingly, admit some justice in this censure ; yet it is obvious that they felt they were acting from absolute necessity ; the child seemed to force their response from them. In one case the child had wept for twenty-four hours before the mother made her the " solemn promise " of her own immortality.

I think we may say that they acted, although perhaps against their better (that is, their rational) judgment, yet on sound intuition, based on empathic understanding of the child's need. For such a need to deny a perceived reality has been shown to be a normal stage in the acceptance of reality.

Negation of reality is a transition phase between ignoring and accepting reality ; the alien and therefore hostile outer world becomes capable of entering consciousness, in spite of " pain," when it is supplied with the minus prefix of negation, i.e., when it is denied (18.b).

By consenting to be parties to the negation of reality, therefore, the mothers were helping the children to accept reality later on ; refusal to consent would have forced the child to escape its " pain " in some way less consonant with its stage of mental development and its individual personality. We may suppose that the later neurotic developments of the little French girl were not unconnected with the fact that her mother was extremely reluctant to help her in the denial of reality.

Thus it seems that the child may weave for himself, and need agreement to help him weave and maintain, a belief in personal immortality. That the self will die is the reality which is only to be entertained when supplied with the minus prefix of negation. It is clear that this stage in the acceptance of reality is not only an ontogenetic one.

Humanity, phylogenetically considered, makes this negation ;[1] indeed, the negation itself has been the source of many of the finest and most impassioned products of the human intellect, in literature, art and architecture. Dr. Malinowski, viewing the development of this faith among men of different levels of culture, has written that

" the spiritual force of this belief (in immortality) not only integrates man's own personality, but is indispensable for the cohesion of the social fabric."[2]

If this belief is really an unbelief, that is to say, a negating stage in the acceptance of reality, we may say with Bishop Blougram, " How can we guard our unbelief, Make it bear fruit to us ? "

That, however, is another question. Whatever humanity may do, the child does not normally remain at this stage ; but he comes to it gradually, and, sometimes through such a crisis as Theodor, Richard and the little French girl went through, he passes gradually on from it. We are able to trace stages both earlier and later.

Some further examples may be given from Richard's record before the behaviour of other children is considered. Before he became so worried for himself personally, he appeared really to believe that he belonged to a chosen people who would escape death :

Richard, aged 5 : 0 (1937)
(First sentence very indistinctly heard :)
R. : Men are meant (made ?) for deaths, aren't they ?
M. : Do you mean sometimes, or always ?
R. : Sometimes, because we won't die, because English don't shoot Englishes.

[1] This is, of course, an over-generalization, even for civilized humanity : it does not apply to Confucians.
[2] B. Malinowski, *The Foundations of Faith and Morals*, p. 61. Possibly Dr. Malinowski may have been playing the part of the mothers. One may suggest it without suggesting hypocrisy, but rather a keen appreciation of the realities of social hygiene.

But four months after the conversation in the bathroom, this idea has been degraded from belief to fantasy. In the course of the long-drawn-out fantasy reported on page 131, Richard (5 : 5) (1937) said,

. . ." thunder is drums of soldiers in the sky—soldiers won't shoot us—because they don't shoot English, only nasty foreign people—we shall go up in the sky if a war comes, so you needn't mind. . . ."
Note by M. : We were in France at the time, and Richard was on the friendliest terms with several French people ; he was also deeply attached to an Austrian maidservant in his own home.

In the conversations of *Stephen, aged 5 : 2* (p. 141), it is apparent that he is going through very much the same stage as Richard, but he (like Ben) tends to associate death mainly with age, number. He is therefore concerned to stress that he belongs to a class of people (in this case males, as opposed to females) who live to be very old. He appears to associate these abilities : to be male, to live long, to have a beard ; and he determines not to shave when he grows up. (Is Stephen acting on a principle of causal magic (*i.e.*, childishly) or in the manner of a statistician who perceives a correlation in phenomena (*i.e.*, like an adult ?). Surely his behaviour might be interpreted in either way. But that is a side issue.)

Thus we see that the negation of death as applying to the self is not always so particularized as to be made applicable only to the individual himself. It may be applied to a whole class to which he belongs. Sometimes that class is the whole class of *children*. This belief sometimes becomes apparent in answers to Stanford-Binet tests. *Mary U.* (11 : 1), when asked the " absurdity " about Christopher Columbus, answered :

" When you're ten years old, I don't see how you could die . . . unless someone kills you."

Another little girl (not a subject for this research, but tested during the same period on the same scale) said :

" Columbus couldn't have died when he was ten, because a boy couldn't have been an enemy."

Schilder and Wechsler (58) report several such statements among the children whom they examined (all clinical cases), thus :

George M. :
   (Q. : Can a child die ?)
   George : No, boys don't die unless they get run over.
Edward G. :
   " I shall not die—when you are old you die. I shall never die. When they get old they die." (But afterwards he says that he will also get old and die.)

Ferenczi has indicated a connection between the stages of acceptance of reality, and the reduction of the " sense of omnipotence " ; he points out that inferiority feelings are not a reduction of the sense of omnipotence into an acceptance of the force of circumstances ; they are a reaction from an exaggerated sense of power, and as such have importance in the production of the negation of reality. My records do not show clearly this connection in particular association with the concept of death. But the home records provide two incidents showing how children deal with anxiety (*a*) in this provisional way, by a negation of reality connected with it, and (*b*) by mastering it in fantasy. And here, with the latest of the home records, the account of them will be concluded.

Example (a)
(*Notes :* Richard has always been small for his age. The children were not aware of observation.)

   Catherine Holland, 8 : 8, Susanna Holland, 6 : 6, and Richard Clement, 5 : 5, are playing together in a garden which opens on to a wood. A public footpath runs through the wood, some distance from the garden.

R. (delightedly) : We'll able (*sic*) to kill it . . . kill him
with a sharp spade . . . chop his legs off and he'll fall down
. . . and I've got a sharp spade . . . I've got a . . . thing.

S. : . . . and I've got a spade. . . . We'll dig a. . . .

R. : And I saw one. . . . Oh, it's really only a person
(disappointedly).

(C. meanwhile is sharpening a stick with a penknife.)

R. : Shall we go out in the woods, and if we really see
one . . . shall we go now ? . . . All right, shall we go ?

S. : Do you think a wooden spade would do any good ?

R. : No.

S. : I'll take an iron spade.

R. : Shall we go now ? The biggest be the leader. I'm
the last. You're the biggest (to C.).

(Observer here notes : " I get the impression that on
second thoughts Richard decides that he doesn't want the
dangerous business of bringing up the rear.")

R. : Well, I'm five. (Then to S., who is 6½ :) *You're only
three ; I'm much older than you. I'm the second oldest ; you're
the last.*

(They set out in procession into the wood, R. in the
middle.)

C. : The youngest *ought* to be in the middle, oughtn't
they ?

(A minute later, all together :)

All : Oh, what's this, what's this ? Oh, look ! (Delighted
cries. Most of their conversation cannot now be heard.)
. . . Oh, look at the wolf ! (The cries of excitement and
joy continue at intervals for about twenty minutes. They
then return to the garden.)

R. (a little plaintively, yet assertive) : I like this play so
much that I want to go on.

C. (firmly) : No, we'll stop now.

(S. gets on the swing and C. pushes her.)

R. (good-naturedly, waving his spade at S.) : I'm going
to kill her, going to kill her. (He laughingly threatens S.,
but is really sad because of the abandonment of the other
game.)

(Later, when R. and M. were getting ready for lunch, C.

and S. having gone home, M. asked about the game, and was able to transcribe the response unobserved :)

R. : We pretended people were ostriches, and we were elephants killing the ostriches. I had my very sharp pen-knife and Susanna had a spade and Catherine hadn't any spade, she had a tent-pole. Oh, I can't do up my shoes ! Everyone else can do up their shoes, but I can't do up my shoes. Shall I make up a story of someone who couldn't do up *any* of their shoes ?

Example (b)

Ben, 10 : 1, and Richard, 6 : 11, with M. just after lunch, R. asked to have *Grimm's Fairy Tales* to read in rest-time, because he likes it very much ; Ben said he did not like Grimm. Then : ˙

Ben : Richard's afraid of witches, and I'm afraid of ghosts.

R. : I'm afraid of witches, and ghosts, and burglars, and *everything*.

B. : Oh, burglars are *real*, you needn't be afraid of *them !* I'd rather like to see a burglar. You needn't be afraid of anything that's in reality. You'd just run down and dial 999 !

(*Note by M. :* Our telephone is not on the dial system.)

CHAPTER XI

THE PROBLEM IN PRACTICE AND THEORY

THE main lines of our exploration, and much of the material collected in the course of it, have now been described, and an attempt has been made to interpret the material in the light of the child's psychological nature and development. It is now time to return to the problems raised in the first chapter, and to consider what light is thrown on them by our findings.

To consider first, questions of every-day practice. It seems clear that, since the idea of death occurs very readily in the fantasies of normal children, there is no reason to lay a ban on those tales of old folklore or of modern fact or fiction which refer to death. Naturally this sanction can have no absolutely general force ; individual children may have peculiar anxieties which demand special care in handling. Tales or attitudes which seek to arouse fear and horror by adding nightmareish circumstance or suggestion to any kind of incident are to be condemned, whether the incident with which these emotions are associated is death or anything else. But the subject of death in itself is not alien to the child's fantasy-thinking, and its introduction into the works of fantasy presented to him may vary and enrich his own conceptions, and so actually prevent them from becoming obsessional and morbid.

We have found little sanction for the grown-up attitude described by Dr. Susan Isaacs, and to some extent exemplified by the Katz parents, which showed the wish to shield the child from all perception or thought of dead things or death. Here again, the individual child has to be considered. Attendant circumstances which would in any case arouse distress, such as violent aggression, obvious danger of disaster or pain, or suggested fears, cannot be presented to the child's mind without tending to arouse anxiety. But there does not seem to be any reason why children should not, for instance, inspect a dead bird on the lawn, or hear of the deaths of people they have known ; nor need the adult be horrified if the child seems rather excited than distressed if allowed to witness scenes (such as the killing of a pig) which many town-bred adults prefer to avoid.

The Katz parents, who at first refused to let their children know that the meat they ate came from animals which had been killed, found later that this knowledge did not disturb the children at all. These children appear to have been quite typical in their unconcern. Nevertheless there do exist children who react somewhat in the way the Katz expected to find normal. When they hear that animals have to be killed to provide meat they may refuse to eat it ; they may become vegetarians from that time onwards for the rest of their lives, without any direct suggestion from other people. The analysis made in Chapter VII of the significance of animals in the development of the concept of death shows what associations may lie behind such a reaction on the child's part, and we should expect to find in such a child a strong, unresolved ambivalence for some member of his family, and a sense of guilt about it, producing some special degree of conflict at the very time when the concept of death was being given more definite shape than it had previously held—for instance, when the change from B category (*infantile ;* median age 5½) to C category (*junior ;* median age 7½) was taking place for that child.

Such an instance did occur, in a very mild form, in one of the subjects of research (Ben Clement). At six years old, Ben asked what animals the different kinds of meat came from, pitied the sheep, pigs and calves, and expressed the

O

view that we ought not to eat meat. His mother told him that there were people who held this view and acted on it, and that if he wished to be a vegetarian he might do as they did, and give up meat altogether. She said it was difficult to know where to draw the line, and gave him no encouragement, though the permission was quite clear. Dinner was served not long after, with pork sausages, which was one of Ben's favourite dishes. While eating some, he asked about the animal it came from. He had a second helping.

When vegetarianism is presented to a child as a normal cultural attitude and practice, and adopted by him in consequence, his behaviour has, of course, quite a different psychological significance from the independent movement towards giving up meat which was made by Ben. Children's reactions to the eating of meat cannot be studied as a psychological phenomenon apart from the attitudes socially suggested to the child. Besides the importance of the general social setting, there is also great significance in the whole psychological setting, so that no reaction can be studied except in relation to that whole, too. The child may identify himself mainly with the animal, or with the slaughterer ; or he may identify himself almost simultaneously with both, and thus either magnify or reduce his conflicting emotions. Complexities are many, potentially, and their expression in behaviour is often difficult to distinguish. It is probably wise to respect (but pay little obvious attention to) children's spontaneous tendencies of refusal to eat meat or to conform to a vegetarian diet, unless the contrary is advised during a general course of psychotherapeutic treatment. Usually the particular reaction to food is only one symptom of a wider conflict, for which it may provide relief. In some cases the reaction may become permanent, and provide an adjustment, which, although not psychologically a complete solution, may not be anti-social. But if the reaction goes with a general picture of neurotic disturbance, or if it is persistent and progressive or exceptionally violent (when, for instance, the person adds more and more foods to the proscribed list, or injures his health by the severity or the character of his denials), a psychological diagnosis is needed.

Another practical question is that of the advisability of young children dissecting dead animals for educational purposes : the question which Dr. Susan Isaacs has raised in her book on *Intellectual Growth in Young Children*. My own observations suggest that most children under the age of eleven years (that is, before the transition to E category is effected) are not *spontaneously* moved to undertake such dissections. Not that they are uninterested in dead bodies of animals, nor that their attention should be drawn away from these objects, but that their interest is mainly of another kind. I believe, from the evidence already given, that these younger children are preoccupied in " working over " the personal, emotional significances of death. To withdraw their attention from this aspect and direct it towards one totally different, namely, the physical dissection of the dead body, may arouse in them, if not active repulsion, at least discomfort or even anxiety.

In some of the accounts of the behaviour of her children at these dissections, Dr. Isaacs does, I think, give us signs of such feelings of discomfort being felt by certain children, and evinced by obvious lack of interest in the activity their companions were engaged in ; and even signs of anxiety are to be found in the records, particularly in the question of one little girl, whether Dr. Isaacs would ever think of doing this to her !

Educational experts may nevertheless support, and have ground for supporting, the practice of zoological dissection by young children. Through education the cultural attitudes of adults are passed on to the child. Civilization depends on the encouragement of the scientific attitude, and the educational reinforcement of the natural desire to know " reality." When a child has expressed spontaneous interest in the functions of the living body, an opening is obviously given for satisfying his curiosity by making use of the body of an animal which has died, and then the impulse to know, supported by the encouragement of the adult, may overcome the impulse to treat the dead body as material only for fantasy, without arousing any undue degree of conflict in the child.

We are, however, from cultural necessity, inclined to value the impulse to know " reality " more highly than the impulse to work over and resolve anxieties in fantasy. Through this attitude the mental health of individuals may be endangered.   A safeguard against it is to await the spontaneous interest of the child.

But these questions of formal education, feeding, and fairy-stories, practical and often important as they are, have not the weight nor the urgency of the main problems of practice that this study touches on, namely, those arising from the child's experience of the death of persons in his own intimate personal circle.   What does death mean to the child then, and what can the grown-up person, related or unrelated to the child, do to ensure that all goes well with him, to recognize his problems when all does not go well, and then to help or cure ?

These are very large questions, which I shall not attempt to answer fully, but certain points which came out during the course of this study have a close bearing upon them, and may be developed further.

First, in this connection, we must bear in mind the fact that the child is liable to feel a strong sense of guilt when a member of his family dies.   This sense of guilt almost certainly will be, from a commonsense point of view, utterly unreasonable.   The behaviour that follows from it may be of the most varied description ; there may be unwonted aggressiveness, with or without excessive excitability, or there may be sullen unsociability and obvious despondence, or there may be an unwonted lack of interest and attention in class, or a degree of forgetfulness of ordinary concerns which calls for remark. There may be unusual reactions in relation to animals, ranging from neurotic fears (phobias) to peculiar sympathies, possibly with refusal to eat animal foods. Different ages will, of course, react in somewhat different ways. The younger child's suffering may arise mainly from a sense of responsibility for the death itself, because in him experience has shaken less the belief in the power of his own wishes to make things happen. The older child may suffer more from a sense of the newly-intolerable burden of minor, cumulative wrong-doings. His clearer conception of time and finality shows him a future in which he cannot atone to the one who has died. In that person's life-time, the *intention* to expiate allowed the child to commit faults fairly happily, and hope to go undetected. Death presents the whole bill, denies the possibility of payment, and refuses the opening of a new account.

Thus the sense of guilt will take different forms, and the reactions to it also will be infinitely various. In some children they may appear so briefly and mildly as to pass unnoticed. Nor can the layman determine with certainty that when such symptoms as I have suggested do appear, they are due to this particular inner reaction. In practice the important thing is to know that a sense of guilt is likely to be present, however unreasonable any real accusation of guilt would be, and to realize that the neurotic symptom may be a result of this, rather than a mode of behaviour to be considered as significant in itself, or treated without relation to the whole situation.

Even when this is recognized, the adult may well be at a loss to know what will most help the child in his difficulty. It is quite common to suppose that giving him the constant companionship of other children of his own age, so as to distract him from his private griefs and preoccupations, is the healthiest and happiest way of solving the problem. For one thing, it is usually the easiest procedure. For another thing, the adult realizes that his own conception of death and his own attitude towards it will not be that of a young child. He tends to feel that he has a deeper sense of the inexorability and bitterness of fate, and, knowing that he may communicate this to one unable to bear the weight of such a burden, he hesitates to make close contact with the child at such a time, however sympathetic he may be about the child's personal loss. He tends to comfort himself with the idea that the child does not realize what it means ; that the permanency of the loss will be transmuted by the child's different sense of time, and that when " never " begins to seem long, the first violence of grief will be already softened.

In so far as the adult recognizes a difference between his own conception of death and that of the young child, he obviously does rightly. But in so far as he sends the child to the companionship of his coevals, and does not offer in any special degree his own society and friendly sympathy, it may be suggested that he does not do so well. Such evidence as I have collected (and it is supported by that of Dr. Ruth Griffiths in her *Study of Imagination in Early Childhood*) goes to show that at such a time the child avoids dealing with the subject of death in his fantasies. That is, he tends to repress the idea ; the sub-complex, as it were, goes rigid within him, and no longer takes its part in the free play of the mind. But he does desire to talk about the fact itself to an adult, and gets relief from objective conversation. I have explained this by supposing that the adult's total rejection of the suggestion of the child's guilt in itself gives the child comfort. The child's sense of guilt is implicitly expressed in his behaviour, and the denial of his guilt is implicitly expressed in the behaviour and attitude of the adult, even without words. The grown-up who feels that comforting words of hers may lead the child into too-deep waters may be right ; there is no call for such words without a clear lead from the child. But if the child is allowed to talk freely about things as he sees them, to ask questions and have them directly answered, then the sorrows he may still feel will tend to be perhaps of their kind no less deep, but devoid of that peculiar painfulness which attends remorse, and the morbidity that marks irrational remorse. He can be given opportunity to talk of the person who has died, and should find that he may express hostility as well as love towards the dead. The suggestion that ambivalent feeling is condoned is perhaps the most active part the adult can take in the cure, but it should be done in such a way that the child does not realize how the adult's suggestion has given him the freedom to express himself. The suggestion may come through a perfectly amoral, " unsentimental " attitude on the adult's part, towards some account of events in the child's past history concerning his relationship with the dead person. She avoids frequent reference to the positive aspects of the emotional relation, and suggests condonation of antagonism : there is, for instance, little reference to " your *dear* mother," and still less to " your *poor dear* mother," " your *darling little baby* brother," etc., but she may say " I suppose he was a nice little chap to play with when he was in a good temper ? " or " Did he ever try to hit you ? "

There may be cases where the sense of guilt does not seem to be strong, but where there is apparent rather a general sense of lack of security, and deep anxiety. Here again, resultant behaviour may be infinitely varied. Such anxiety, perhaps by unconsciously equating the death-separation with the separation of birth, may take the form of absolutely irrational fears of water, or of suffocation, or of enclosed spaces.

In connection with all such reactions, one has to remember that the death of someone loved arouses not only sorrow at the loss, but also desire to be not separated, and hence to be dead, too. But then a deep conflict ensues, for there is desire for death and at the same time aversion to the idea of dying, being dead, being impotent (according to the main significance death may have for the individual who is suffering this conflict). So there is a desire to be dead, and at the same time a fear of the fulfilment of the desire. The more strongly the sufferer is imbued with the sense that what he wills comes true, and the more he desires death, the deeper will be this fear.

Through the different equations of life after death with life before birth, or with birth itself, a fear of enclosed spaces (claustrophobia), or of the dark, or of being left alone, or of large empty spaces (agoraphobia) may be the result in a young child of the death of someone he loves. Here again, the treatment is very similar (in those cases which do not call for or cannot receive complete psychotherapeutic treatment) to that suggested for the child who suffers most from a sense of guilt. The symptom as such should not have primary attention, but the child should be offered in a special degree the comfort of sympathetic adult company, so that his sense of general insecurity and his anxiety may be relieved. Ultimately this will happen through the partial substitution of the image of the lost guardian by the image of another or others who care for the child. The substituted image may in some cases be composite, though this is less likely to happen with the younger children.

In recent psychological work on children's problems so much stress has been laid on the approach to the child through his fantasies, that the suggestions here made, laying weight rather on the more direct approach and the conscious aspect of things, may seem both unorthodox and old-fashioned. It may, however, be defended without any attack on the present orthodox practice of child-psycho-therapy. Those children who can immediately make use of the new facts (such as the death of a member of their family) in their fantasies, and whose general behaviour remains normal, may well be left to work over their problems in this way. With children under the mental age of five this may very likely happen. But participation in childish fantasies by an adult, if it is meant to direct mental life away from morbidity and into healthier channels, is best left to the psychologist trained in play-therapy. Many children whose mental balance is temporarily upset have no chance of receiving such specialist attention. The adult untrained in psychotherapy may still help them ; this is the point I have stressed, because I believe it is not generally recognized. The child who is suffering from a sense of guilt or of insecurity may find comfort and be brought into healthier touch with reality by having the chance to talk to a sympathetic grown-up person about the facts of the situation, or consciously to express his fantasies or describe his dreams, rather than by the solitary weaving of fantasies, or the companionship of his contemporaries only.

Guilt and anxiety are in some degree a normal reaction to the experience of others' death, which social and religious conventions are designed to reduce, and which time normally diminishes. But if they persist unchanged for months, or if they give rise to severe or recurring obsessional or hysterical symptoms, then there is obviously need for special treatment.

The obsessional or hysterical symptoms point to the fact that some memory or sub-complex is being repressed. The act of repression is itself commonly unconscious ; in adult cases it seems to be usually so. But with children the boundaries between conscious and unconscious are less clearly defined, and repression may itself be a conscious act, and may even be expressed in movements whose purpose is discernible by an observer. A child who wants to repress the thought of death or the memory of someone who has died, may run away when the subject is mentioned, or put his hands over his ears, or absolutely refuse to take part in any conversation which touches on the subject. He may refuse to look at anything intimately associated with the dead person. Or he may shut his eyes or ears by mental inhibitions, turning to some other interest in his thoughts or his play. These things he may do either consciously or unconsciously (though the two kinds of reaction will not be identical).

Such behaviour may appear " quite natural." But when such repression is the child's main form of reaction to the new experience it is a danger-signal. The realization and acceptance by the mind of the fact of general and inevitable death is a stage on the road of mental development which each civilized man must pass through if he is to leave mental infancy behind. Death is essentially an " external reality " on the conceptual level. The mind builds up a pattern from recognized reality, into which it casts all new experience, and by which it shapes all ego-activity. The pattern moulds the perception of experience, but also the experience, if it does not fit into the prepared mould, in the normal process of growth affects and changes the pattern. If a particular experience which does not fit the earlier patterning of reality is rejected, instead of bringing about a change of the pattern, then the whole development of the process of reality-perception is adversely affected.

Yet rejection is not an entirely morbid process. Harmful things must be rejected by the body, and also in its own way by the mind. What, however, cannot be rejected, consistently with mental or physical health, is the belief in the harmful thing's existence. In the very *raison d'être* of mental activity there exists, therefore, this conflict : the mind must grant perceptual admission to what the body needs to reject. We must recognize what will harm us ; that is, we must open our minds to it, welcome it there, weave it securely into the reality pattern which is intimately ours. But what the body must reject, parallel impulses or emotions in the mind also reject ; the conflict is not one between mind and body, but is fully represented within the mind.

The safety, health and development of body and mind depend on this rejection *following after cognition*, and not taking the place of cognition or of its normal effects. To take an example familiar to the psychologist : the chick must recognize the existence of the bad-tasting, poisonous caterpillar as such, before he habitually ceases to pay attention to it in his search for caterpillar-food. In terms of mental life, repression, which is equivalent to rejection of poisonous things as such, must occur after the object of thought or emotion (be it a *thing*, an *imago*, or a complex memory) has been perceived as real, existent, and personally distasteful. The baby sees and knows the " bad mother " or the denying, empty bottle, before he represses the memory so as to enjoy to its maximum the good, generous one.

By the body and by the emotional impulses most closely connected with physical impulses, all that involves death must be utterly rejected. Death of the self implies the most absolute negation of the prospect of attaining the ends of those physical and emotional impulses. The realization that all men are mortal is essentially a summation of everything that instinct leads the living being to reject.[1]

When the growing mind, therefore, reaches the stage when it can, and indeed must, conceive of death, the conflict which is always present in consciousness sharpens ; each side brings up all its forces, and the edge of battle joins.

If, then, the idea of death, instead of being assimilated into the whole pattern of the intellect, moulding that pattern anew and then sinking to comparative quiescence, is as a result of emotional impulses rejected from it and assimilated instead with ideas which have, after full cognitive activity,

---

[1] The Freudian death-instinct complicates this picture, mainly because Freud does not, I think, make clear under what conditions the death-instinct externalizes itself through the musculature (*i.e.*, death is physically rejected from the self) and under what conditions it acts in the primitive, passive way, making death welcome. The statement in the text in any case remains true of " the living being," though admittedly the limitation reminds us of the story of the centenarian who attributed his longevity to eating an onion a day. " My father," said a bereaved young man, " also ate an onion a day." " Ah ! " said the centenarian, " but I expect he didn't keep it up long enough ! " Both the *libido* and the death-instinct lead the *living* being to reject death. And although throughout life we are dying beings as well as living ones, the preponderance during the developmental period is in life's favour.

been repressed in accordance with cultural demands, then this is a sign that the personality may, in the course of social development, be split violently and permanently along the wrong lines. All adult personalities are to some extent split along the lines Id-Ego, Conscious-Unconscious, with which Freudian psychology has made us familiar. But the personality which refuses to accept passage through the ego-structure for the realization of death, will be split along lines which are not consistent with the development of civilization, and there will be set up in him a perpetual conflict between reality as he sees it, and the reality which is a basis for the society he lives in.

Such acutely repressive behaviour in a child therefore raises fears of mental disintegration in later life, more particularly if the repressed material finds no indirect outlet in neurotic symptoms. It suggests that later on there may be an assimilation of perceptual as well as conceptual reality with the things unrecognized and repressed, and the patient will become unable to distinguish even between visible forms, audible sounds, etc., and his own fantasies. In addition to the refusal to accept the reality of death, he may then return to other modes of thought normal in infancy, with which such a non-realization is in keeping.

Children do not only reach the stage where the idea of death must be assimilated, when experience presents them with the actual loss of someone loved. It is a stage which everyone must go through, whatever the accidents of their experience. In the chapter on children's definitions of "dead," I have attempted to show what earlier developments the child passes through on his way to this stage. We found that for most children the eighth year is a turning-point, and that by the twelfth year the assimilation is commonly completed.

There may be in some persons a predisposition to refuse to assimilate unpleasant ideas in general. Mental activity, however, is so deeply founded on this ability in all human beings, and even the earliest developments of perception would be so impeded without it, that we have little ground for assuming the existence of *innate* differences, in this respect, so extreme as of themselves to lead some individuals inevitably to mental disintegration as a consequence. When such a general predisposition is found, it must rather be assumed that it arises through fostering circumstances in early childhood. Apart from this, there may be in some children a particularly strong rejection of the idea of death, owing to special conditions of character and emotional experience. In such children the repressive process may take place, and disintegration may follow from it, without any immediate tragic stimulus in individual experience. But if a child, in the critical years when the idea of death presents itself, suffers a special loss, or is concerned in a sudden or shocking tragedy, and reacts to it by acute repression of the whole idea of death or the dead, then the form of the experience combined with the particular stage of the child's development would appear to be largely responsible for the form of his reaction, and it is not to be attributed solely to predisposition. On the relative frequency of such a case-history there is no material available.

The child in either case needs care and cure, whether he refuses to accept the idea of death because he has a specially strong predisposition to find it intolerable, or because particular experience has made it more than normally painful at the critical stage. The task is no light one, and it is well if special psychotherapy is available, for the direct approach is no use in such cases.

The layman, however, probably does much to prevent this kind of morbid reaction if she avoids early suggestion of repression of the idea of death, by her own words or example.

In discussing previously the cases of young children who denied that they themselves would ever die, and who were supported in this attitude by their mothers, it was suggested that the mothers behaved wisely in agreeing with the child. This may seem to be a contradiction of the statement that the adult should not suggest or encourage repression of the idea of death in the child.

But it is not a direct contradiction. Freud has shown that explicit negation of an unpleasant thing is not synonymous with repression of the idea, but is a stage in the acceptance of it. So the child who says " I shall never die " is actually occupied in weaving the thought of death into his pattern of reality.

Moreover, the behaviour of these children was the less likely to lead to morbid development later, in that it was transient ; the moment was critical, but the child's mind did not dwell there with any permanence. As a stage in the acceptance of reality, negation is not a danger ; danger may arise if development is arrested at this stage.

These are the contributions to the practical care and handling of children which the present study suggests. What is its contribution to psychological theory ? That has already been made in the course of the exposition itself, but may be summarized here again. The main propositions are these :

(1) That the idea of death *occurs readily in children's fantasy thinking.* (Chapter III.)

(2) That the idea arises as *a response to suggestions of grief and fear,* the grief being frequently associated by the child with loss or *separation* and the fear with *aggressive intrusion.* (Chapter III.)

(3) That fantasy about death is commonly found together with *talion* ideas (retaliation, reparation) ; the talion idea, however, appears to be as much *a mode of mental functioning* as a content of thought. It is a mode *according to which fantasy-themes oscillate as to the aspect they present,* somewhat as the aspect of perceived objects may oscillate when held in the forefront of attention. That such oscillation

occurs in connection with the process of identification. (Chapter III.)

(4) That *genetically* the idea develops according to a certain form similar to that described by Piaget for the development of the child's conceptual thought in general : namely, from a stage of ignorance (with egocentric characteristics), through an intermediate stage (C), here characterized as being homocentric and concerned mainly with cultural-symbolic aspects of the idea, to a mature stage (E) which shows objectivity and wider generalization. (Chapters IV and VI.)

(5) That the idea of death *becomes emotionally charged through being brought into association with memory-complexes relating to birth* (*and pre-natal life*) *and to hostility and aggression.* This emotional charge and the gradual assimilation of it appear to correspond to stage C. (Chapter VII.)

(6) That in the death-aggression complex, *animals* play an important part, as being the legitimate victims of human aggression both by striking and by eating. (Chapter VII.)

(7) That *the development of conscious logic and rational science*, and their final dominance, are closely connected with the development of the concept of death. When the hate-aspect of erotism has been repressed, the realization of the power-lessness of the individual to avert death from the loved object proves to him that he is not omnipotent—that is, that he has not magical powers, and that natural law prevails over human will.

The *first step* in the development of logic and science is therefore *the dominance of love* in consciousness ; the *second* is *the recognition of the inevitability of death.*

The *third step* occurs when *death is associated with the self.* In the attempt to avoid this association the child proceeds from transduction (or induction based on ubiquity of causation) to true induction and deduction based on the uniformity of natural laws. (Chapter VIII.)

(8) That the *magical thinking about death* which gives rise to spontaneous childish *beliefs* or hypotheses, commonly originates in an identification of death with birth or pre-natal life, while the identification of death with results of aggression tends to be expressed in *fantasy.* It is suggested that the

former originates in pre-Œdipal erotism and the latter in erotism complicated by ambivalence and rivalry. (Chapter IX.)

(9) That children may pass through a stage when they seek to allay anxiety aroused by the association of death with the self by denying that they will die. That this is a method of rendering the painful idea capable of entering consciousness ; a transition phase towards the acceptance of reality which may, if necessary, be supported by the adult. (Chapter X.)

Two further points remain to be noted : first, that the child, in giving up his belief in his magical powers and accepting the dominance of logic and reason, may not attach absolute finality to death. The essential thing is that he admits his inability to escape it, in so far as it is socially or objectively presented to him as a fact. Secondly, it must be realized that in relinquishing his magical potency, the child also casts off a load of responsibility and in many cases a deep sense of guilt, in respect of the deaths of others.

Only gradually, however, do the results of new conceptions of reality affect the deeper unconscious mind.

During the present century, psycho-analysis has abundantly demonstrated how impulses which function nakedly among babies and primitive peoples are still functioning under cover in the minds of civilized men. The old theories of recapitulation are out of date, and the psychologist does not now suppose that the individual lives through each stage of the history of the race in due order. But in observing the development of the concept of death in individual children, one seems to see re-enacted a later stage of human history than that wherein psycho-analysis has hitherto found its more illuminating parallels. Here are mirrored the mental struggles and the great intellectual advances which marked those ages when the religions of the civilized world were first developed, and the Hellenes opened up the true path of science.

APPENDIX TO CHAPTER I

STORY-COMPLETION RESPONSES FROM CHILDREN WHOSE MENTAL
CONDITION APPEARS TO BE PATHOLOGICAL

(For test, see p. 16.)

(1) *ERNEST V., aged 9 : 1. Mental age 6 : 6.*
(This record was taken by a colleague. Ernest was seen
at a Special School for Mental Defectives. His I.Q. was 72.
The following notes were made : " Lively, friendly boy ;
chatters incessantly. Admits to minor delinquencies without
apparent sense of guilt. Gets too little sleep and too much
stimulation.")

1. 'Cos the others might hit him.
2. 'It 'im on the 'ear'ole.
3. 'Cos 'e wouldn't eat 'is dinner.
4. Was angry 'cos the boy kept asking for money.
6. Showed shop where he took apples and oranges—
Ronnie Morris takes oranges from the shop with me.

7a. 'Cos 'e did all those stories, morning.
7b. 'Cos 'e ain't got no ma or pa. My father died
Saturday ; I went to wake 'im up and 'e was dead—in
bed—but 'e wasn't asleep 'cos 'e was dead ; I know when
'e's asleep 'cos 'e snores like a pig—'ad a lovely funeral,
horses and carts but they go too slow. My mother takes me
anywhere now—we're going to Newcastle where there are
soldiers to shoot you. I don't want 'im back now 'e's dead.

8a. 'Cos 'e liked to stop at 'ome and play with toys—'is
teacher 'it 'im on the 'ead.

8b. Someone in the bed might do something to his eyes—
would bash into something, happened to kid up the road
—cut 'er 'ead off and she came to dinner next day. Two
hundred fire engines went down our street last night.

9. A toy—railway set.

10. Be little—go out in a pram and let someone push him.

11. Spend it on toys, what I'm going to do, railway set. Lot of milk and biscuits to eat.

(2) *PETER V., aged 8 : 2. Mental age 6 : 2*
(At the time this test was given, Peter had been having play therapy at a Child Guidance Clinic for several months and was reported from school to be much improved. E. had only had him as patient for a short time. His parents lived a life of constant disagreement : a separation was imminent. Peter remained in touch with E. for about nine months subsequently to this test, and has shown signs of achieving comparatively normal emotional development. Poor physique and intelligence are handicaps.)

2. Smacked 'em.

3. Oh, because the . . . because he was very naughty —the boy.

4. The reason was father—father was—he quarrelled, because—this is very naughty—because he could not do as he's told.

5. She said, " Don't go out, father, don't go out " (Peter shouts this in a strange voice).

E. : And did he go ?
Peter : Yes. (Peter meanwhile is building with bricks, and here he speaks about his building) : This is going to be a big beer-shop. It's going to fall down somewhere. I don't know where it's going to fall. (He sings and whistles.) Don't look yet. Not till it's made. I've got a lot to do yet.

6. A toy ; motor-car. It's a motor-car, but it's very strong.

7a. He thought about Jesus. He say, " Oo, would you come in my house, please." (P. says this in a squeaky voice.)
E. : And did he ?
Peter : No.

7b. Mummy. Mummy smacked 'im on the face and made 'im cry again.

8a. Jesus. Jesus again. (All in a loud whisper.)

8b. Oh, because of the bang of the church went dong—eh ?

9. Sweets.

10. Please, no ! (Peter shouts.)

E. : Wanted to grow up ?

Peter : Yes. Turn into a big man. But his father said No. So he did.

E. : Was he angry with his father for saying No ?

Peter : Yes.

E. : When he grew up, what did he do ?

Peter : Sling him in the bang. I'm not finished yet (his building).

E. (in agreement) : No.

Peter : Say, Oh yes, you are. (He demands a quarrel.)

E. : And what will you do when you're a man ?

Peter : Climb up the pub.

E. : On to the roof?

Peter : Yes.

(3) *CHARLIE (aged about 7 : 0 ; mental age about the same as Peter's.)*

(This boy's mother had been for some time in a mental home. He was a boisterous, aggressive boy, of good physique ; intelligence dull but not defective ; manner so lively as to make him appear comparatively intelligent. He had been attending a clinic for group-play for over a year.)

1. Because the little boy was naughty, and when it was over the little boy never went up and a master told the little boy to go down and he never took no notice so a policeman came to school and said to the master, " Anyone been naughty . . ." . . . said he would put the little boy in prison—no food—nothing—won't see his mother any more. Then the little boy promised to be good ; then he went out and got lost—went on a charabanc—fell off—broke his head—the doctor couldn't fix his head on, so . . .

2. They got lost and so the little boy didn't know his way home—he went to the police—they said, " What you come here for ? "—" Because I got lost " (that was right, wasn't it ?). The policeman chained him up, put him in the coal cellar. His mother came—the door was locked—she was

crying—rats and mouses—and that was finished, because the mother got sick and ill, and that's the end.

3. (Laugh) I don't know. *You* tell *me* a story.

4. The mother went to the police and she asked the police, the father's very angry, and the police never took no notice, he was deaf, so he went to hospital, he had a tummy-ache, belly-ache, went home, went to bed, felt very hungry. . . .

5. He (She?) was very miserable. So they all went to bed, and they feeled sick and when they got up in the morning they fell down on the floor, dead, so he phoned up, and they put him ('im, 'em?) in a police car. . . .

7*a*. About his mother.

7*b*. I don't know that.

(Charlie has come to the test from the play-room, and is anxious to go back. We therefore rush on to the fairy.)

9. A toy.

10. Grow up—be a man.

E. : What would he do when he was a man?

C. : Build houses and paint houses and go to the Troc and be a waiter.

BIBLIOGRAPHICAL LIST

Numbers preceding the entries are those used for reference in the text. Some works referred to in the text have not been given numbers, as the alphabetical order of the list makes reference sufficiently simple.

Some works have been listed here only because reference has been made to them in the text (for example, Lewis Carroll, *Alice in Wonderland*) ; others have been listed although no reference has been made to them in the text, because they were found relevant and particularly interesting or significant (for example, Flugel's *Psycho-analysis of the Family*, Saurat's *The End of Fear*, Celine's *Voyage au Bout de la Nuit*, Zuckermann's *Social Life of Monkeys and Apes*).

Omissions from the list are not only due to carelessness or ignorance (for which apology must be made), but in some cases to the fact that the author's name already appears in the list, and his contribution is so considerable that only particular references or works particularly relevant can be noted. For example, valuable material may be found scattered throughout the works of Freud, Frazer, Malinowski, and the books of the Old and New Testament.

Some obvious omissions are due to the difficulty of consulting libraries, including one's own, in war time. Entries for Catullus Fenichel, Spearman, Surrey, are among those which have suffered for this reason.

The list might easily be extended ; its limitation is necessarily somewhat arbitrary. An effort has been made to include all scientific studies of the development of the idea of death in the (normal, civilized) individual ; the total found was not large. On the subject of suicide, and on ideas and customs relating to death in savages, a much more extensive bibliography would have been possible : further lists may be found in books on those subjects listed here.

Some studies of psychoses have been included, because of the reversal of normal development which they may illustrate.

The following shortenings of journal titles have been used :

213

Am.J.Orthopsych.	American Journal of Orthopsychiatry
Am.J.Psychiat.	American Journal of Psychiatry
Am.J.Soc.	American Journal of Sociology
Arch. de Psych.	Archives de Psychologie (Geneva)
B.J.P.	British Journal of Psychology
B.J.Ed.P.	British Journal of Educational Psychology
I.J.P.A.	International Journal of Psycho-analysis
J.Ab.Soc.P.	Journal of Abnormal and Social Psychology
J.Soc.Psych.	Journal of Sociology and Psychology
Psychoan. Rev.	Psychoanalytic Review
Rev.fr.psychoan.	Revue française psychoanalytique

ALEXANDER, F. "The Need for Punishment and the Death Instinct" : *I.J.P.A.*, x, 1929.

1. BARRIE, J. M. *Peter Pan, or the Boy who wouldn't Grow Up.*
2. BARTLETT, F. C. *Remembering.*
3. BECKER, H. "The Sorrow of Bereavement" : *J.Ab.Soc.P.*, xxvii, 1932–3.
   BENDANN, E. *Death Customs.*
   BENDER, L. See SCHILDER.
4. BENEDICT, R. F. "Magic" (article in *Encyc. of the Social Sciences*).
   BERGLER, E. "Psycho-analysis of the Uncanny" : *I.J.P.A.*, 1934.
5. BIBLE, THE.
   (a) The Book of the Revelation of S. John the Divine, chs. xx, xxi.
   (b) The First Epistle of S. Paul to the Corinthians, ch. xv, v. 21. ("For since by man came death, by man came also the resurrection of the dead.")
   (c) Ecclesiastes, ch. xii, vv. 5–7. ("And desire shall fail, because man goeth to his long home, and the mourners go about the streets.")
6. BINET, A.
   (a) For tests. See BURT, TERMAN.
   (b) *L'Étude experimentale de l'Intelligence.*
7. BIRRING, E. "Psychology of the Ideas of Death in Paranoiac Schizophrenia" : *Psychan. Rev.*, xx, 1933.
8. BOSWELL, J. *Life of Samuel Johnson*, vol. i (1791).
9. BOVET, P. *The Child's Religion* (English trans., 1928), p. 31.
   BROMBERG. See SCHILDER.
10. BROWNING, R. B. *Poetical Works.* "Bishop Blougram's Apology."

11. BÜHLER, K. *The Mental Development of the Child.*
12. BUNYAN, J. *The Pilgrim's Progress* (1678).
13. BURT, C. *Mental and Scholastic Tests*, p. 27.
14. BUTLER, S. *The Way of all Flesh*, ch. lxxix.
    BYRON, N. G. G., LORD. *Poems.* " The Destruction of Sennacherib."
15. CARROLL, LEWIS (DODGSON, C.). *Alice in Wonderland* and *Alice Through the Looking-glass.* Postscripta. 1876.
    CASEY, R. P. " The Psychoanalytic Study of Religion " : *J.Ab.Soc.P.*, 33, iv. 1938.
16. CATULLUS,—(Poem beginning : " Multas per gentes atque multa per aequora vectus.")
    CÉLINE, L-F. *Une Voyage au Bout de la Nuit.*
    CHADWICK, M. " Notes upon the Fear of Death " : *I.J.P.A.*, 1929.
17. DE MORGAN, W. *Joseph Vance* (p. 19, 1929 ed.).
    DE QUINCEY, T. *Autobiographic Sketches*, ch. i.
    DURKHEIM, E.
    (*a*) *The Elementary Forms of the Religious Life.*
    (*b*) *Le Suicide.*
    ELIOT, T. D. " A Step towards the Social Psychology of Bereavement " : *J.Ab.Soc.P.*, xxvii, 1932–3.
    FEDDEN, R. *Suicide.*
    FENICHEL, O. " The Pregenital Antecedents of the Œdipus Complex."
18. FERENCZI, S.
    (*a*) *Stages in the Development of the Sense of Reality* (1913).
    (*b*) *Further Contributions to Psycho-analysis* (1926). *The Problem of the Acceptance of Unpleasant Ideas.* (Quotation from Freud, S., Negation, *Imago*, 1925.)
    FLUGEL, J. C. *Psycho-analytic Study of the Family.*
    FOXE, A. N. " Omnipotence as a Defence " : *Psychoan. Rev.*, xxv, iv.
19. FRAZER, J. G.
    (*a*) *The Belief in Immortality and the Worship of the Dead* (1913).
        (i) p. 193–4. (ii) p. 195. (iii) p. 35.
    (*b*) *The Golden Bough.*
20. FREUD, A.
    (*a*) " On the Theory of Analysis of Children " : *I.J.P.A.*, x, 1929.
    (*b*) *The Ego and the Mechanisms of Defence* (1937), pp. 37, 38.

21. FREUD, S.
    (a) *Introductory Lectures on Psycho-analysis* (1922).
    (b) *New Introductory Lectures on Psycho-analysis* (1933).
            (i) p. 157. (ii) p. 130.
    (c) *The Ego and the Id.*
    (d) *Beyond the Pleasure Principle.*
    (e) *The Future of an Illusion.*
    (f) Collected Papers (particularly :)
            II. *A Child is Beaten.*
            III. *From the History of an Infantile Neurosis.*
                 A Case of Obsessional Neurosis (p. 368).
            IV. *Analysis of a Phobia in a 5-year-old Boy.*
                 The Theme of the Three Caskets.
                 The Uncanny.
                 Thoughts for the Times on War and Death.
                 Mourning and Melancholia.
    (g) *Totem and Tabu.*
    (h) See FERENCZI.
22. GOSSE, E. *Father and Son.* (Quotations from pp. 114, 254, 1925 ed.)
23. GRIFFITHS, R. *A Study of Imagination in Early Childhood.*
    (i) p. 141 ff.
24. GRIMM, J. *Fairy Tales (Kinder und Hausmärchen).*
25. HASTINGS, J. " Death " (article in the *Encyc. of Religion and Ethics*).
    HARNIK, J. " One Component of the Fear of Death in Early Infancy " : *I.J.P.A.*, xi, 1930.
    HEIDEGGER, M. *Sein und Zeit* (quoted Schilder).
26. HEMANS, F. *Poems.* " Casabianca."
    HENDERSON, D. and GILLESPIE, R. D. *Textbook of Psychiatry,* p. 198, 3rd ed., 1933.
27. HERMANN, I. " A Study of G. T. Fechner " (abstract, *Psycho-an. Rev.,* xxiv, 4, 1937).
28. HOCART, A. M. " Death Customs " (article in the *Encyc. of Social Sciences*).
29. HOUSMAN, A. E.
    (a) *A Shropshire Lad.*
    (b) *Last Poems.*
30. HOFFMAN, H. *The English Struwwelpeter.* Nos. 3 and 7.
    HUGHES, R. *A High Wind in Jamaica (or, The Innocent Voyage).*
31. HUME, D. *An Inquiry concerning Human Understanding.* IV, ii.
32. ISAACS, N. " Children's ' Why ' Questions." (Appendix to S. Isaacs' work 33 (a) next page.)

33. ISAACS, S.
   (a) *Intellectual Growth in Young Children.*
         (i) p. 160. (ii) p. 359. (iii) p. 204. (iv) p. 183.
   (b) *Social Development of Young Children.*
         (i) p. 161.
JAMES, W. *Varieties of Religious Experience.*
JERSILD, A. T., MARKEY and JERSILD. " Children's Dreams,
   Fears, Wishes, etc." : *Columbia Child Development Mono-
   graphs*, No. 12, 1933.
JOHNSON, S. See BOSWELL.
34. JONES, E. Papers on Psycho-analysis (1938 ed.), in particular:
   (a) *The Theory of Symbolism.*
   (b) *The Significance of the Grandfather* (p. 520).
   (c) *The Phantasy of the Reversal of Generations.*
   (d) " The Phallic Phase " : *I.J.P.A.*, xiv, 1, 1933.
JUNG, C. G. Psychology of the Unconscious.
35. KATZ, D. and R. *Conversations with Children* (Eng. trans.,
   1936).
         (i) p. 251 ff. (ii) No. 59. (iii) Nos. 33 and 53.
KEATS, J. *Poems.* " La Belle Dame sans Merci."
36. KLEIN, M.
   " Symbol-formation in Ego-development " : *I.J.P.A.*, xi,
   1930.
   Psycho-analysis of Children (1932).
KOFFKA, K. *The Growth of the Mind* (p. 341–2).
37. KÖHLER, W. *The Mentality of Apes.*
KRAEPELIN, E. *Dementia Praecox* (trans. Barclay, 1919).
42. LECONTE DE LISLE, C. R. " Les Elfes " (*Oxford Book of French
   Verse*, 299).
43. LÉVY-BRUHL, L. *Primitive Mentality.*
44. LEWIS, M. M. " The Beginning and Early Functions of
   Questions " : *B.J.Ed.P.*, viii, 1938.
45. LOVELACE, R. *Poems.* " To Anthea from Prison."
46. LOWIE, R. *Primitive Religion.*
47. MACAULAY, T. B. (LORD). *Essays and Lays of Ancient Rome.*
   " Horatius."
48. MALINOWSKI, B.
   (a) *Baloma ; the Spirits of the Dead in the Trobriand Islands.*
         1916. (i) p. 367.
   (b) *The Foundations of Faith and Morals.* 1936. (i) p. 61.
   (c) See OGDEN and RICHARDS.
MANSON, R. and PEAR, T. H. " The Testimony of Conversation " : *B.J.P.*, January, 1937.

49. MARETT, R. R. *Faith, Hope and Charity in Primitive Religion.*
    1932.
            (i) p. 41. (ii) p. 25. (iii) p. 51.
    MENNINGER, K.   " Psychoanalytic Aspects of Suicide " :
    I.J.P.A., xiv, 3.
50. MIDDLETON, W. C. " Some Reactions towards Death among
    College Students " : *J.Ab.Soc.P.*, xxxi, 2, 1936.
    MILTON, J. *Poems.* " Lycidas."
51. MORGENSTERN, S.   " La Pensée Magique chez l'Enfant " :
    Rev.fr.psychoan., vii, 1, 1937. (i) p. 112.
    MURPHY, G. " Types of Word Association in Dementia
    Praecox, Manic-depressives, and Normal Persons": *A.J.
    Psychiat.*, II, iv, 1923.
    NEW STATESMAN, THE.   Controversy between Stephen
    Spender and the organization called Mass-observation
    (C. Madge, T. Harrisson). This reference has been lost.
    OGDEN, C. K. and RICHARDS, I. *The Meaning of Meaning.*
    With an Appendix by B. Malinowski.
    OPLER, M. " Further Comparisons of Anthropological Data
    bearing on the Solution of a Psychological Problem " :
    J.Soc.Psych., IX, 4. November, 1938.
52. PEARSON, K. *The Ethic of Freethought* (p. 13).
53. PIAGET, J.
    (*a*) *The Language and Thought of the Child.*
            (i) p. 175. (ii) p. 178.
    (*b*) *The Child's Conception of Causality.*
            (i) p. 127. (ii) pp. 240, 241. (iii) p. 267.
    (*c*) *The Child's Conception of the World.*
            (i) p. 151 ff. (ii) p. 139. (iii) p. 136.
54. PLATO, *Phædo*, (trans. H. Cary, Everyman ed.) (i) p. 203
    (ii) p. 149. See also *The Meno* p. 99.
    POE, E. A. *Poems.* " Annabel Lee."
    RANK, O. *The Trauma of Birth.*
55. RASMUSSEN, V.
    (*a*) *Child Psychology.*
            (i) I, 22. (ii) II, 36–42.
    (*b*) *Diary of a Child's Life.*
            (i) under date 1.9.17.   (ii) 27.8.17.   (iii) 7.8.19
            and 15.9.19.
    REIK, T. *The Unknown Murderer.*
    RICKMAN, J. " Unbearable Ideas " : *Am.J.Psychiat.*, 1937.
    RIVERS, W. H. R. *The Primitive Conception of Death.* Essay in
    Psychology and Ethnology, 1926.

SAURAT, D. *The End of Fear*, 1939.
56. SCHILDER, P. and BENDER, L. " Suicidal Preoccupations in Children " : *Am.J.Orthopsych.*, vii, 1937.
57. SCHILDER, P. and BROMBERG.
   (*a*) " Death and Dying " : *Psychoan. Rev.*, xx, 1933.
   (*b*) " The Attitude of Psychoneurotics towards Death " : *Psychoan. Rev.*, xxiii, 1936.
58. SCHILDER, P. and WECHSLER, D. " The Attitudes of Children towards Death " : *J.Ab.Soc.P.*, xlv, 1934.
   SCHMIDEBERG, M. " The Role of Psychotic Mechanisms in Cultural Development " : *I.J.P.A.*, xi, 1930.
59. SEARL, M. N. " The Psychology of Screaming " : *I.J.P.A.*, 1933, xiv, ii.
60. SHAKESPEARE, W.
   (*a*) *Sonnets*. Nos. xii and xx.
   (*b*) *Hamlet* (in Ophelia's grave, V, i).
   (*c*) *Romeo and Juliet* (in the tomb, V, 3).
   (*d*) *Coriolanus*, I, 3.
61. SPEARMAN, C. *The Nature of Intelligence and the Principles of Cognition.*
   (i) p. . (ii) p. 297.
62. STEKEL, W. *Conditions of Nervous Anxiety.* (i) ch. xxvii.
63. STERBA, E. " Analyse d'un cas de phobie des chiens " : *Rev.fr.psychoan.*, vii, 4, 1934 (trans. from *Z.f.Psychoan.Päd.*, 1933).
64. STERN, W. *Psychology of Childhood* (trans. A. Barwell, 1930).
   (i) ch. xxviii.
65. STOUT, G. and MACE, C. *Manual of Psychology.*
66. SULLY, J. *Studies of Childhood* (1895).
   (i) p. 240. (ii) pp. 248, 460, 475–6. (iii) p. 478. (iv) p. 224. (v) pp. 453–4. (vi) p. 105 ff. (vii) p. 444.
67. SURREY, THE EARL OF. The elegy for Clere is reprinted in Ward's *English Poets*, Vol. I.
68. TACITUS, P. C. *Agricola.* XLVI.
69. TERMAN, L. *The Measurement of Intelligence.* (i) p. 118 and pp. 221–4.
70. TERMAN, L. and MERRILL, M. *Measuring Intelligence* (1937, Eng. ed.).
   (i) p. 101. (ii) p. 114. (iii) pp. 302–3. (iv) p. 303 (n.).

71. THOMAS, M. Méthode des Histoires à compléter pour le
dépistage des complexes enfantins. *Archives de Psychologie
(Geneva)*, *xxvi*. *1937*.
        (i) p. 253. (ii) p. 233.
THOULESS, R. H. *Introduction to the Psychology of Religion.*
72. TRAHERNE, T. *Centuries of Meditations.* (i) Century III, 1–3.
73. VALENTINE, C. N. " A Study of the Beginnings and
Significance of Play in Infancy " : *B.J.Ed.Psych.*, vii, 3,
1938.
74. ZILBOORG, G. " Considerations on Suicide with Particular
Reference to that of the Young " : *Am.J.Orthopsych.*, vii,
1937.
ZUCKERMAN, S. *The Social Life of Monkeys and Apes.*

INDEX

Page numbers in italics indicate a home-record entry

behaviour relative to Death, *See* Death

Chivalry, the relation of sex and death in the culture of, 67–8

" Clarissa " (an extraneous H.R. child), *152–3*, 153

Closure, operative in fantasy, 23, 38–9

Correlation, between chronological and mental age of subjects, 84n., 85 (table), 98 ; between response-categories, *See* " Dead " and chronological age, 83n., 84 (table), 98 ; and mental age, 83n., 84 (table), 98

Cowper, W., 76

Cruelty, I in children, to animals, examples of apparent, *120*, *122–4*, *126–8*, *130* ; examples of, in fantasy, *190*, *191* ; motives of apparent, 120, 124–5, 126, 127, 128, 129–30 ; social reaction to, 128, 130 ; Sully on, 126 ; *See* Animals, Birds'-nesting, Aggression ; II to children, in religious teaching, 80

D

Dante, 68

David (friend of H.R. children), 120, 125 ; loves wasps as victims, *123–4*, *143*

" Dead," children's definitions of, 32, Ch. V *seriatim*, 146 ; classification of, in categories A–E, 81–3 ; parallels with, in Home Records, 101, 105, 119 ; relation of chron. age with, 83, 84 (table), 87 ; relation of mental age with, 83, 84 (table), 86, 88, 90, 92–9 ; influence of relevant experience on, 86 ; influence of home teaching on, 96–99 ; insertion of, in intelligence test, 27, *See* Age, Death

Dead, untouchableness of the, *120*, *121*, 124–5, *129 and n.*, 179

Death, actual experience of, the effect of the, of self, 72n. ; of relatives, on the development of the concept of, 86 and n., on children's fantasies and behaviour, 1–2, 55–62, *102–3*, 106, *118*, 155, 196–202 ; on adults, 70, 79–80, 144, 6 ; of people not necessarily relatives, on children, 63, *97*, *117*, *119*, *139*, *169* ; on adults, 68, 73–4 ; of animals, on children, 193, *See* Animals ; -complex, 3–4 ; denial of (belief in immortality), Ch. X *seriatim*, 6, 65, 73, 75–7 ; and development of logic, 160–2 ; in relation to a group, 187–9 ; in relation to self, 6, 184–9, 205–6, 208, 159 ; socially expressed, 6, 159, 187 ; *See* Heaven, Logic, Reality ; desire for, 199 ; for parent's (lover's) company in, 136, 138, 142–5 ; discovery of, 4, Ch. VI ; euphemisms for, 36 ; fear of, anxiety about, x, xi, 1–2, 33, 63, 67–80, 199 ; felt by child, of his mother's, 136, *137–8*, *140*, *141*, 145n., *152*, 157, *181–2* ; of his own, 48, 59–60, 62, *138*, *141*, *143–4*, *156*, *157–9* (table), 160–2, *180*, Ch. X *seriatim*, 205–6, 207–8 ; felt by adults, Ch. IV *seriatim*, as witness their attitude to children, 35, 71–2 ; neurotic reactions to, 69–71, *See* Psychoneurotic Behaviour ; science as relief for, 78n. ; sex as relief for, sexual aberrations as origin of, 67–9 ; identified with absence, birth, effect of old age, punishment, *See* separate entries, result of aggression, separation, sleep, the self, departure, journey, *See* Departure, deprivation of food, *See* Food, details of dissolution, 96 ; illness, hospital, 94–5 ; impotence, 95–6 ;

mental conflict between acceptance and, 202, sharpened in case of death-concept, 203–4 ; is morbid if occurring before acceptance has functioned, 202 ; then leads to abnormal type of dissociation, peculiar systems of reality not typical of the adult, 204–5 ; zoological dissection as an education in, 195–6

Rebirth, reincarnation, examples of children's belief in, 46, 54, 169, 171–4 ; of disbelief in, 173 (2) ; as occurring within the same family, 171, 176–7 ; in oscillations of fantasy, 54–5, 62

Reincarnation, *See* Rebirth

Religion, motives of primitive, 124 ; social function of, in relation to death, 6, 78–80, 187, *See* Agnosticism, Deity, Heaven, Hell

Religious teaching, 162 ; Christian, on death, 74, 75–6, 77, 78 ; of children, 17th-19th centuries, 74–76 ; subsequently, 77 ; influence of, on definitions of " dead," 96–8, 99, 130, 131 ; on H.R. subjects, 15–16 ; instances of, 130–133, 174–5

Reparation, 53, 54, 59, 181 ; derived from Talion idea, 53–5, *See* Retaliation

Resistance, 9, 19 ; circumvention of, 9–13 ; as an index of identification, 20–22 ; to avowal of death impulses by adults, 65

Resurrection, the place of the idea of, in the cumulative oscillations of talion fantasy, 55 ; occurs in the recorded fantasy of children, 121–2 (Catherine), 132 (quoted by Isaacs), 131–2 (quoted by Rasmussen)

Retaliation, in children's fantasies, 48–62 ; derived from oscillations of fantasy, 49–55 ; at

different levels of social behaviour, 53 ; an ethical procedure, 53, 54 ; based on identification, 53 ; in death-aggression complex, 147

Reversal of generations, 169, 171

" Richard Clement," 14, 15, 101, 121–2, 127, 129 ; shows egocentric characteristics, 105 ; enjoys killing, 120 ; comments on accession of Edward VIII, *117* ; drowns kitten, 122 ; kills cat in fantasy and repairs it, *122–23* ; kills bee, 123 ; kills ants, *123* ; kills an earwig, *123* ; " loves killing things," *124* ; kills worms and says it doesn't matter, *124* ; " likes being cruel to animals," *124* ; motives of, 125 ; fond of a dog, 125 ; killing by treading, 128–9 ; asks about the dead mouse, *129* ; " up in the sky if war comes," *131* ; departed—dead ? *135* ; indifference to anticipated death of m., *137* ; sorrow only comprehensible if death is of a child's m., *137* ; finds substitute for grandm., *138* ; the old become children, *169*, 170n. ; life brings return to womb, *169*, 170 ; complies but disagrees with his brother on reincarnation, *173*, *174* ; interest in Heaven, 174, 175 ; on existence and location of God, *175* ; critical anxiety, 183 ; fear of death, *185* ; assertion of immortality of the English, *187*, *188* ; further negation of reality, *190* ; joins in aggressive animal play, *189–191* ; reaction from omnipotence to inferiority, *191* ; likes Grimm, 191 ; afraid of everything, *191*

Robertson Smith, W., 148

Rousseau, J.-J., 5 ; Institut (Geneva), 16, 43

Printed and bound by CPI Group (UK) Ltd, Croydon, CR0 4YY

01/11/2024

01782629-0006